tao paths

harmony

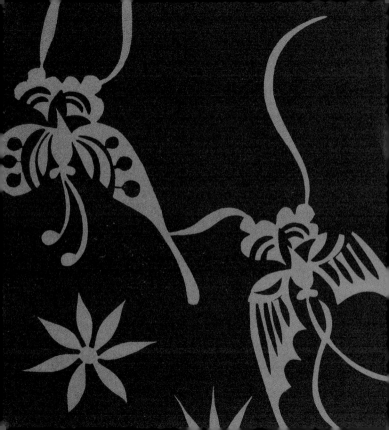

tao paths

harmony

**Andrews McMeel
Publishing**

Kansas City

Contents

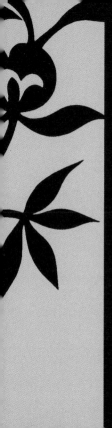

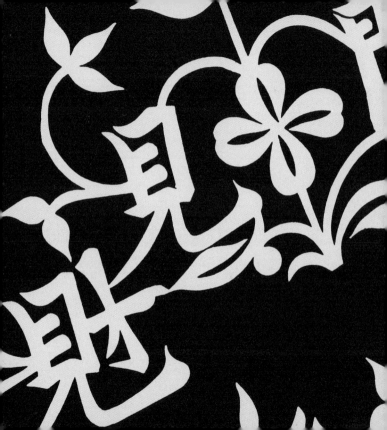

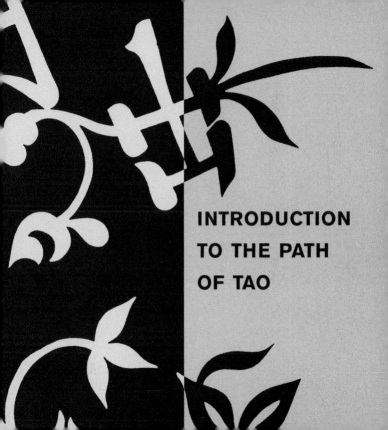

INTRODUCTION
TO THE PATH
OF TAO

Spirituality, on the Path of Tao, is seen as a tangible, even physical thing. Followers of Tao believe that spirituality is connected to *chi*, the life force. It is this basic life force that enables us to experience spiritual insight and feel a connectedness to All That Is, the Tao itself.

Whether we are practicing meditation, *chi kung*, or studying the words of the ancient masters, we are utilizing this life force to enable us to see more clearly into our own lives. In this way we can begin transforming ourselves from our low, often troubled states into higher, more refined stages of spiritual life.

The early sages of Tao, such as Lao Tzu and Chuang Tzu, used images from Nature or metaphors of the great sage rulers to educate us in how to become more balanced, more harmonious, more in touch with our essential spiritual nature. Indeed, the character for master, Tzu, is also the character used for child.

Lao Tzu said:
"In concentrating your spirit and practicing flexibility, can you become like a newborn infant?"

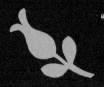

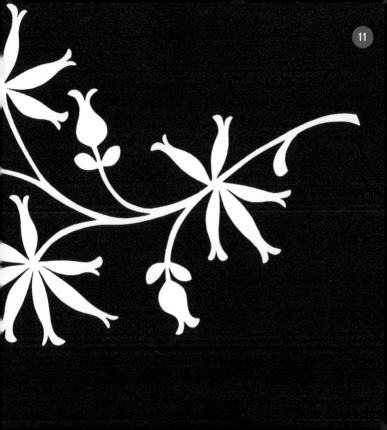

The Path of Tao is one of wholeness, balance, and harmony. It began eight thousand years ago in China yet continues today wherever anyone follows these basic principles. It is less a religion and more a philosophy. It is a way to work with change rather than against it.

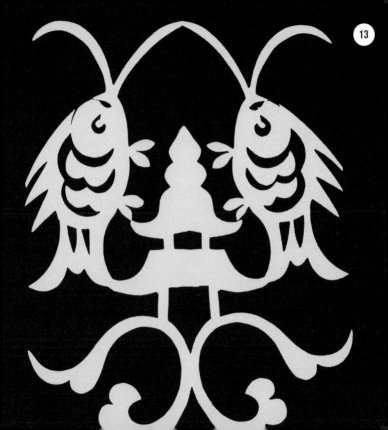

The Path of Tao is that of least resistance, of going with the flow of Nature (*wu wei*). It uses the metaphor of water, which adapts itself to the shape of whatever container it finds the low places and, though soft and yielding, can, over time, cut its way through solid rock.

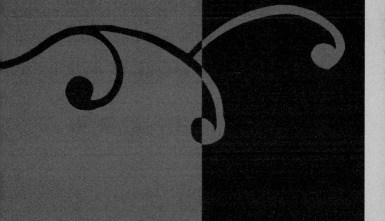

Lao Tzu, the great ancient sage of Tao, said that the Path of Tao is one of seeing simplicity in the complicated and achieving greatness in small things. It is a Path that respects and even honors the Value of Worthlessness and the Wisdom of Foolishness.

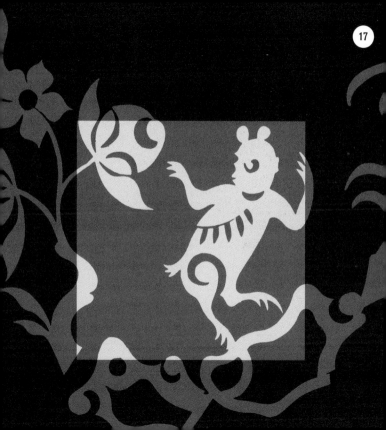

Chuang Tzu, the other great sage of Tao, says:
"Those who follow the Tao are strong in body, clear of mind, and sharp of sight and hearing. They do not fill their mind with anxieties and are flexible in adjusting to external conditions."

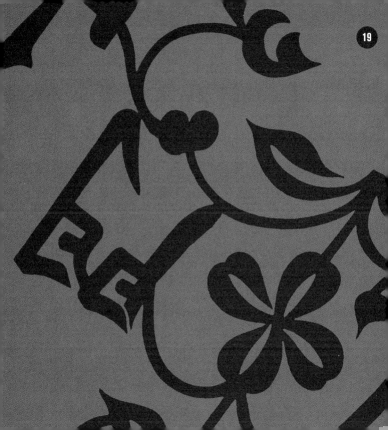

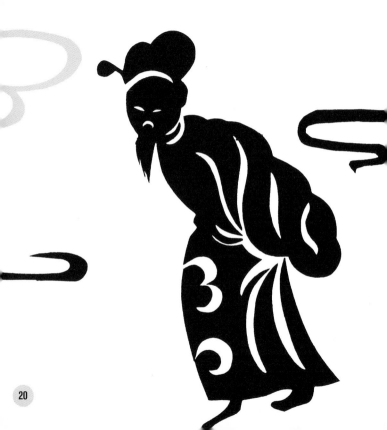

The Path of Tao is a way of life followed by the peasant, the farmer, the gentleman philosopher, and the artist. It is a way of deep reflection and of learning from nature which is considered the highest teacher.

The Path of Tao offers us a simple, practical way of being and living, a way of comporting ourselves on our journey between birth and death and beyond.

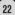

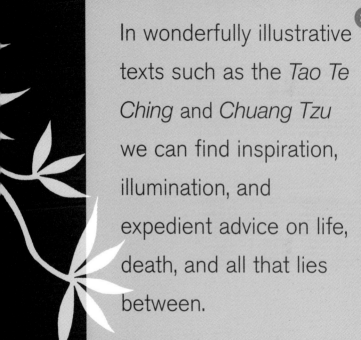

In wonderfully illustrative texts such as the *Tao Te Ching* and *Chuang Tzu* we can find inspiration, illumination, and expedient advice on life, death, and all that lies between.

In Chinese medicine practices, we can find cure and comfort for many modern and not-so-modern ills and complaints. The practices of *chi kung* and *tai chi* can give us ways to stabilize and balance our bodies, allowing us to lead long-lasting and healthy lives. Taoist advice on sexuality and relationships can guide us gracefully through the difficult labyrinth of human sexuality.

And through Taoist spiritual and meditation practices we may finally arrive at that precious point of power described in the Taoist tradition as Returning to the One—the source of our own being as well as being-ness itself.

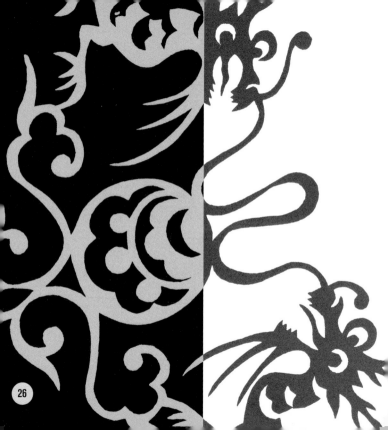

The Tao Paths series offers quotes gleaned from the traditional Taoist works as well as jewels of wisdom from contemporary Taoist masters. Alongside these words of wisdom you will find stories to delight, mystify, and enlighten you to the deep layers of Taoist thought and practice.

Covering a wide range of Taoist tradition we will explore the ways in which the ancient sages as well as the modern masters have given us tools and practices to plumb the depths of our being and reunite us with our eternal source, the Tao itself.

Tao Paths, Love will teach how to maintain healthy relationships—emotionally, psychologically, and sexually; to study the relationship between ourselves and the natural world around us and the infinite depth of our own internal world.

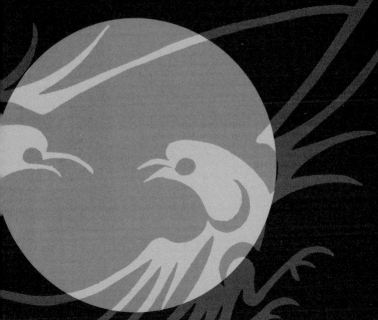

Tao Paths, Harmony will teach us how to be at one with the world around us.

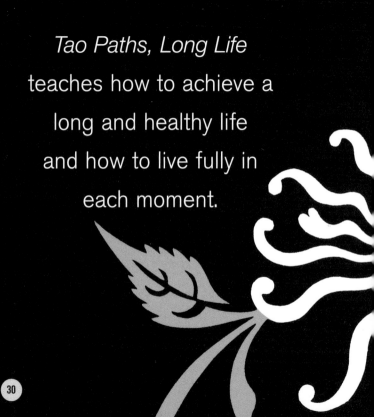

Tao Paths, Long Life teaches how to achieve a long and healthy life and how to live fully in each moment.

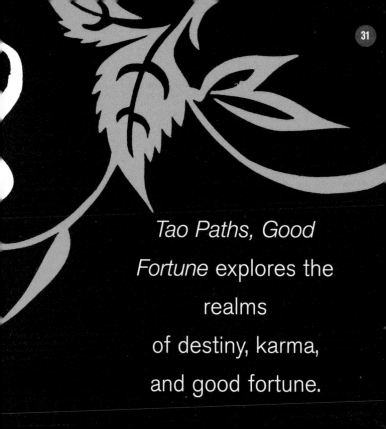

Tao Paths, Good Fortune explores the realms of destiny, karma, and good fortune.

The problems of today are real and profound. They often seem unresolvable, and call for something that can be applied to everyday life. The Path of Tao offers not a way out, but a way through. Its advice and wisdom is real, and eminently applicable, regardless of race, religion, or gender.

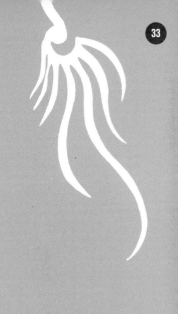

What the ancient men and women of Tao learned through countless years of observation and practice can be just as useful today as it was in the time of the legendary Yellow Emperor.

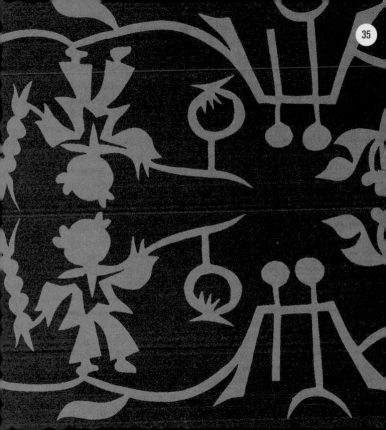

Remember that the Path of Tao is not just an ancient, foreign, mystical path; it is a cross-cultural, nonsexist, practical, even scientific way of viewing the world and our place within it. Its practices and philosophy work on many different levels—physical, emotional, psychological, and spiritual.

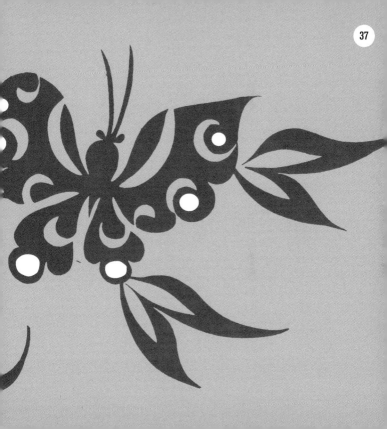

The beauty of the Path of Tao is that there is nothing to join, no vows to take, no special naming or clothing style to follow.

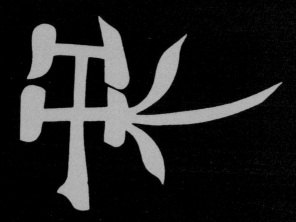

There is no reason to give up your own religion or culture to benefit from the wisdom of Tao. Its teachings can be applied on many different levels in many different circumstances.

Today, in China, there are temples of Taoism, a religious form of Tao (*tao jio*), complete with priests, liturgy and rituals. But the original philosophical form of Taoism (*tao jia*) was intended as a way of life. It is this form of Taoism that we will be working with.

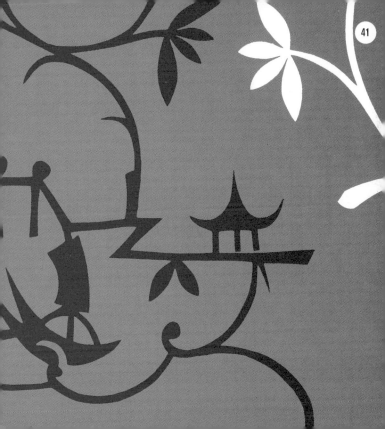

Though the roots of Taoism go back thousands of years, the knowledge gleaned over the centuries can be just as helpful for the modern world as in the Tang Dynasty. Taoism guides us onto the path of least resistance, helps us find a way to work with the currents of change and renewal, and allows us to feel our sense of connection to the sacred.

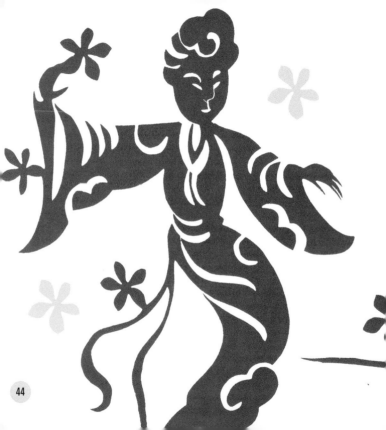

You will meet many strange and wonderful characters in these pages—from the lofty wisdom of Lao Tzu to the often ridiculous metaphors of Chuang Tzu to the down-to-earth tales of Lieh Tzu.

In between you will meet hunchbacks, cripples, lords and servants, wise sages, and foolish seekers after Truth. But pay attention, you may meet yourself here.

In this book you will meet sages, rascals, kings, and peasants. You will hear the wisdom of thousands of years of Taoist masters. It is up to you to take

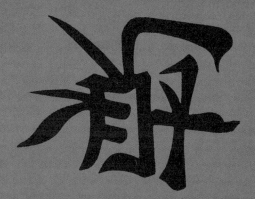

their words and make them a part of your own life. The words and ideas offered by the ancient ones are simple and clear.

Come then on this
journey of self-discovery
and self-cultivation.
There is no need to
change your religion or
spiritual path.

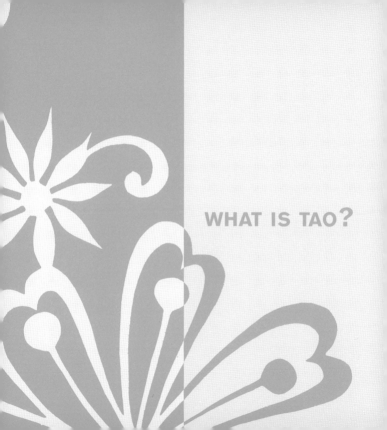

WHAT IS TAO?

The term Tao, pronounced *"Dao,"* is used to describe the indescribable, to put into words what is wordless, to give sound to the great silence. It is our source, our path, and our end as it is our beginning.

The Chinese word *Tao* is made up of two characters. One means to follow or to run and the other is a human face. In this way it can be translated as a person moving along a path.

It can also be thought of as the Path or Way itself.

Tao is the universal pageant of the constellations. It is the budding of each new leaf in the spring. It is life and death and all that falls between, an undying cycle of change and renewal.

While Tao is not personalized it sustains all of creation, giving life and supporting that life to all living beings—human, plant, animal, water, even the very rock foundation of the earth itself. And, in the end, when we have shrugged off this mortal coil, we return to the bosom of undifferentiated consciousness, the Tao.

In the beginning of all things there was a great void. This was called Primordial Chaos. It contained nothing that could be named. Then, from the Chaos came existence, from which we were born. Our goal, as mystical seekers, is to return to the Primordial. This is called Entering the Tao.

The Path of Tao is
dedicated to discovering
the dance of the cosmos
in the passing of each
season as well as the
passing of each precious
moment in our lives.

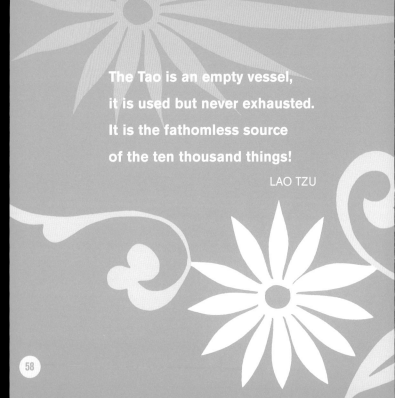

The Tao is an empty vessel,
it is used but never exhausted.
It is the fathomless source
of the ten thousand things!

LAO TZU

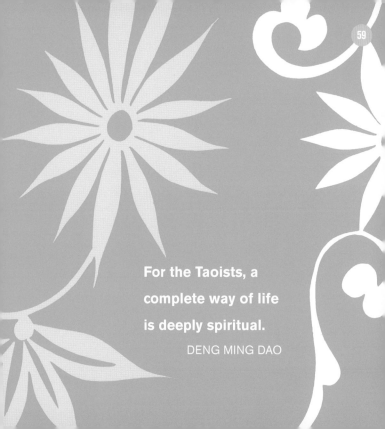

**For the Taoists, a
complete way of life
is deeply spiritual.**

DENG MING DAO

By connecting to our eternal
self, by finding a way back to
our source, we can experience
a sense of peace, of safety,
and of harmony with the
world around us.

**A dedicated Taoist is one who
seeks to live as closely in
accord as possible with nature.**

JOHN BLOFELD

Taoists believe that Nature is alive, that all living
things are composed of primal energy or *chi*.
It is when we allow ourselves to connect with
the outer world of Nature and with our own
inner nature that we can feel balanced,
whole, and connected to all of life.

Try to spend time each day simply being—
being still, being quiet, being breathed. In this way
you will be better able to hear the music of the
spheres and feel the touch of your guiding spirits.

Many cultures speak of a time when humans communicated with animals, of a time when there was no distinction between humans and the natural world. We are now separated

from the world of Nature, our own birthright.
By allowing our own natural instincts to guide
us we can become again like ancient peoples,
at one with all life.

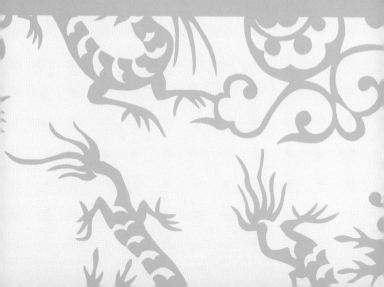

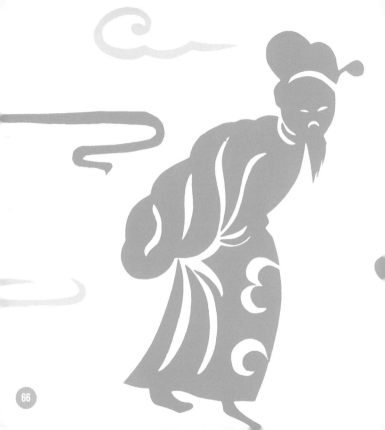

Pen Lo had bred horses for his king for many years. Now he was getting old and the king asked him if there was anyone in his family who would be able to take over for him.

Pen Lo said, "You can tell a good horse by looking at its muscles and appearance. But the best horses are the ones that cannot be judged by their appearance only. You must be able to see their inner nature. No one in my family has this ability.

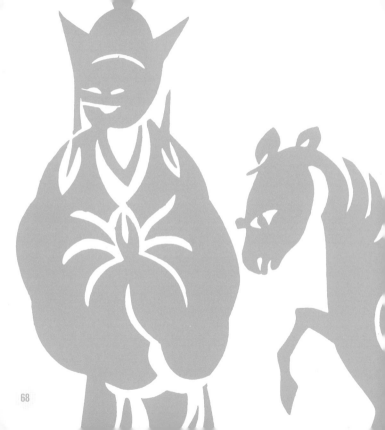

But I do know of one man who might be able to help you. He is a poor man who hauls wood and vegetables for a living. But he has the ability to differentiate the superior horse from the merely great."

The king was happy then and sent for the man and asked him to find him a special horse. The man was gone for three months and then sent word to the king that he had found such a horse.

"What kind of horse is it?" asked the king.

"It is a yellow mare," was the answer.

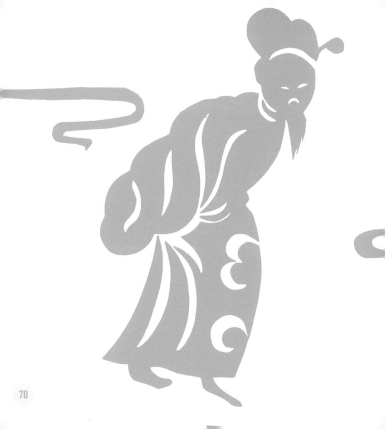

So the king sent for the horse and it turned out to be a black stallion. The king was angry then and sent for Pen Lo. "This man you sent to me knows nothing about horses," he said. "He cannot even tell a mare from a stallion, never mind yellow from black."

Pen Lo's face lit up. "Ah," he said. "It is even better than I had hoped. His ability is now ten thousand times greater than mine. He has completely transcended judging a horse by its appearance and sees only its inner nature.

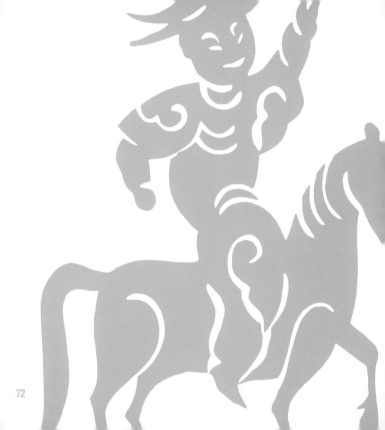

When he looks at the horse he does not see a male or female or what color it is but looks instead to its very essence. In this way he can see the potential for greatness in a horse."

Indeed, when he had sent for the horse, the king found that it was the greatest horse he had ever seen.

LIEH TZU

Try to look beyond what is apparent and instead focus on what is hidden. Look behind the present moment and see what is eternal. Forget about what is obvious and cast your gaze on what is just below the surface.

Wake up and smell the miraculous
fragrance of your own life and of all
the life forms around you! The very
richness of existence is contained in
all that you know and are, and all
that you wish to know and be.
Accept it into your consciousness,
your own expression of the Tao.

Something mysteriously formed,
Born before heaven and earth.
In the silence and the void,
Standing alone and unchanging,
Ever present and in motion.
Perhaps it is the mother of ten
thousand things.
I do not know its name.
Call it Tao.

LAO TZU

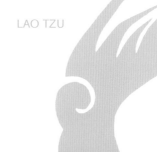

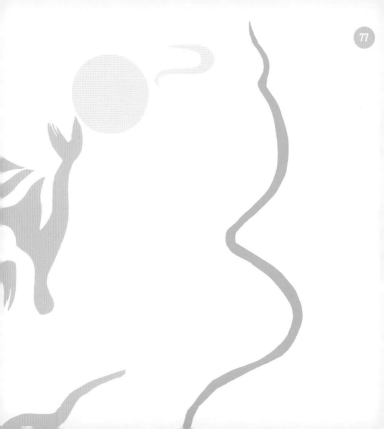

The Tao is a certain kind of order, and this kind of order is not quite what we call order when we arrange everything geometrically in boxes or rows. That is a very crude kind of order, but when you look at a bamboo plant, it is perfectly obvious that the plant has order.

ALAN WATTS

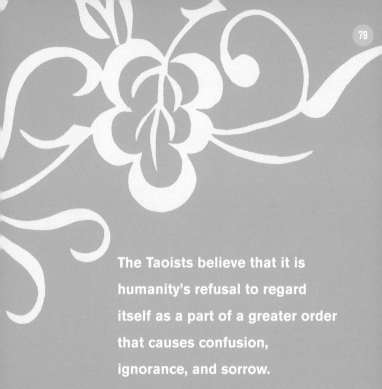

The Taoists believe that it is
humanity's refusal to regard
itself as a part of a greater order
that causes confusion,
ignorance, and sorrow.

DENG MING DAO

In considering the ultimate nature of the Way to be inherently beyond the bounds of human conception, ancient Taoists sought traces of the Way in the patterns of events taking place in the natural world, the social world, and the inner world of the individual psyche.

THOMAS CLEARY

The Way is eternal, infinite
and right in front of us.
By looking for it somewhere
else we lose the Way.

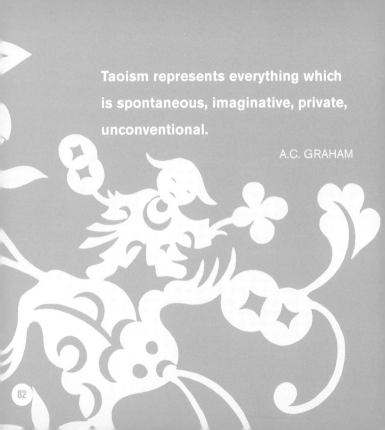

Taoism represents everything which is spontaneous, imaginative, private, unconventional.

A.C. GRAHAM

Taoists believe in the divinity, the special, and deep down holiness of each individual, including themselves.

The Tao that can be put
into words is not the
true and eternal Tao.

LAO TZU

It has been said that words can actually get in the way of true communication. It is when we leave the world of words behind and enter deeply into the world of spirit that we can truly be said to be saying something.

"What is the Tao?" asked the student.

The Master replied, "I will tell you when you have drunk all the waters of the West River in one gulp."

"I have already drunk the waters of the West River in one gulp," answered the clever student.

"Then," said the Master, "I have already answered your question."

CHUANG TZU

When we have the true sense of the Tao, of the real knowledge and wisdom, we will be able to make the right decisions in our lives.

MANTAK CHIA

It is when we let go of our attempts to control the world around us and yield to the ongoing expression of Nature and our place in it that we can find true freedom.

Shun asked the Master, "Can you possess the Tao?"

"You can't possess even your own body," answered the Master. "How could you possess the Tao?"

"If I don't possess my own body," asked Shun, "then who does?"

"It has been lent to you by heaven and earth. Life itself is not your possession. Tao is a harmony heaven and earth has lent you. You don't possess your own nature or your own destiny. They have been lent to you by heaven and earth. Your children and their children are not your possession. They are as molted insect skins, lent to you by heaven and earth.

So when you walk you don't know where you are going, when you stop you don't know where you are, when you eat you don't know what it is that you are eating. The *chi* of heaven and earth is so much stronger than yours but even it can't possess the Tao."

CHUANG TZU

The Tao is the Way, but it is
also the Source, the Journey,
the Traveler, and the Goal.

HUA CHING NI

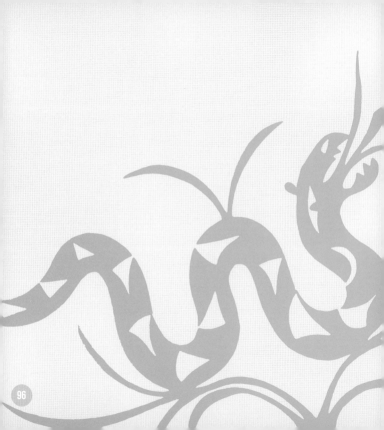

Change is inescapable. We have no control over it. The only thing we have control over is our own responses to the changes life has to offer.

Because the Tao cannot be grasped by our mundane senses, it is futile for us to use ordinary perception to discover the Tao.

LIEH TZU

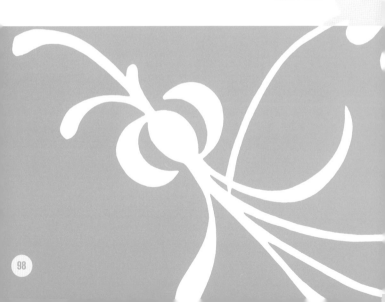

...the only way to know the Tao is to
experience its power in practice,
not just to talk about it in theory.

DANIEL P. REID

Tao is the face we had before we were born.

You look at it and it is not seen, it is called the Formless. You listen to it and it is not heard, it is called the Soundless. You grasp it and it is not held, it is called the Intangible.

LAO TZU

The Taoist seeks to dig deep
under all the layers of
cultural and psychological silt
that has accumulated in us
humans over the millennia
and bring from it the shining
pearl that lies beneath.

Once Chuang Tzu dreamed that he was a
butterfly, flitting merrily through the flowers.
When he awoke he was not sure if he was
Chuang Tzu who had dreamed he was a
butterfly or a butterfly that was dreaming
he was Chuang Tzu!

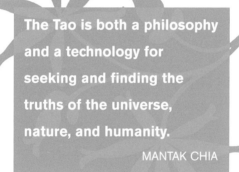

The Tao is both a philosophy and a technology for seeking and finding the truths of the universe, nature, and humanity.

MANTAK CHIA

Any spiritual path worth its salt must be able to address all three levels of existence, the physical, the mental, and the spiritual, in a way that is real and practical as well as transcendent.

The word Tao means the way,
the way of nature and the
universe, or the path of
natural reality. It also refers to
a way in which we can open
our minds to learn more about
the world, our spiritual paths,
and ourselves.

MANTAK CHIA

By paying attention only to what you can see with your eyes you will miss seeing what is really there. It is only by seeing with the inner eye that one can see the true Way.

Why is the fundamental path of life not widely practiced or widely understood? The wise miss it by being superior, the unwise miss it by not being high enough to reach it. Everyone eats and drinks, but there are only a few who know the real taste.

HUA CHING NI

**Keep to non-being yet hold on to being
and perfection is yours in an instant.**

LU SZU-HSING

To enter the Path of Tao means simply to be the best, the most sincere, the most devout, the most understanding, the most patient, the most conscious person we can be.
And as such we can truly call ourselves followers of the grand and divine Way.

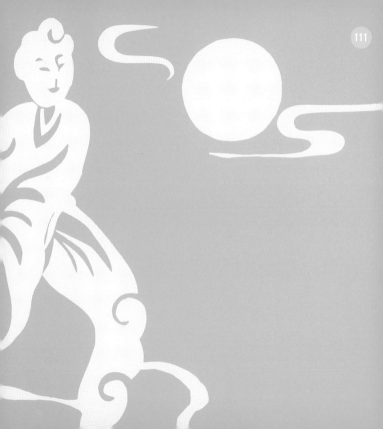

What gives life to all creation and is itself inexhaustible –that is Tao.

JOSEPH NEEDHAM

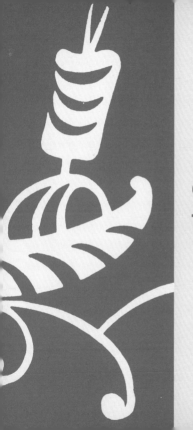

GOING WITH
THE FLOW

Lao Tzu uses the image of water many times in his work the *Tao Te Ching*. The sage or realized person is said to be humble, flexible, present, invisible, and open to each unfolding moment.

It is the image of water—which takes whatever shape it finds itself contained in, that flows downhill and resides in the lowest places, that is in itself colorless, and that has the patience to carve itself through solid rock—that most fully describes such a person.

It is in the concept of *wu wei* (not doing), that we find the idea of not going against the flow of Nature, of not spitting into the wind. Of course in order to be aware of just what the natural flow is at any one time one must become ever more sensitive, ever more attuned to each moment as it is born out of the previous one and flows into the next. What is appropriate action in one instance may not be appropriate in the next.

The Path of Tao is not one of complete submission and surrender. Remember, the most powerful and deadly martial arts in the world were developed by men and women of Tao.

Rather it is the ability to know when to be aggressive and when to surrender. And sometimes it is the knowledge that the best thing to do in the given situation is to do nothing. And in this way, as Chuang Tzu tells us, nothing is left undone.

Under heaven nothing
is more soft and
yielding than water.
Yet for attacking the
solid and strong,
nothing is better;
It has no equal.

LAO TZU.

The fluidity of water is not
the result of any effort on
the part of water, but in its
natural property.

CHUANG TZU

By taking on the characteristics of water—flexibility, patience, adaptability, and clarity—we can ourselves become eternal.

Those who comprehend the Tao are not focusing only on themselves; they are also connected to the world.

HUAINANZI

The alternation of joy
and sorrow, life and
death, is itself the Way,
and we run counter to it
when we strive to
perpetuate joy and life.

A.C. GRAHAM

A Taoist conserves his energy
by easily according with
and adapting himself to
each situation.

JOHN BLOFELD

Wu wei is a kind of perception of the currents of any situation and our place in it. *Wu wei* is the opposite of *yu wei*, or action with useless effort. It is coupled with spontaneity and a deep awareness of what is happening in any situation, allowing us to discern whether it would be better to act or not to act. It is a kind of spontaneity which, as Clare Waltham says, cannot be captured, only fostered.

Wu wei is an attitude, an approach to life itself. When we become sensitive to the current of change all around us we will be able to make intelligent decisions at all times, using the innate wisdom of our bodies and energy systems as well as our minds.

By learning to relax and discover the intrinsic flow of events that contain and are contained by our lives we can reach some measure of security and perhaps even wisdom.

How do we learn this? Perhaps by following the advice of A.C. Graham, translator of Chaung Tzu, when he writes: "If he wishes to return to the Way he must discard knowledge, cease to make distinctions, refuse to impose his will and his principles on nature, recover the spontaneity of the newborn child, allow his actions to be 'so of themselves' they are like physical processes."

The true character of *wu wei* is not mere inactivity but perfect action—because it is to act without activity.

THOMAS MERTON

By softening, by yielding, by listening deeply to the currents of change that go on all about us at all times, we can ourselves become a part of the ongoing panorama of life.

She who practices the Way does less and less every day, does less and goes on doing less until she reaches the point where she does nothing, yet there is nothing that is not done.

CHUANG TZU

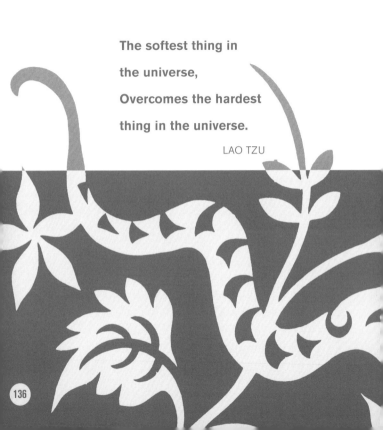

The softest thing in
the universe,
Overcomes the hardest
thing in the universe.

LAO TZU

Those who have attained the Way can respond to the unexpected without fear and can escape from trouble when they encounter it.

WEN TZU

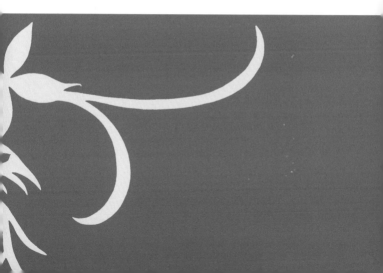

To be able to deal with problems before they become problems is the highest attainment.

Those who are good at walking
leave no tracks;
Those who are good at speaking
make no mistakes;
Those who are good at calculating
need no counters;
Those who are good at closing
things need no key,
Yet what they close cannot
be opened.

LAO TZU

Once Confucius was looking down into a gorge where a great waterfall crashed down to a huge roiling chasm so violent that no fish, tortoises, or even alligators could survive there. Suddenly he noticed an old man appear to tumble over the falls into the maelstrom. Horrified, Confucius, along with several of his disciples, ran downstream in hope of saving the poor unfortunate, only to find the old man strolling merrily along the bank, singing to himself.

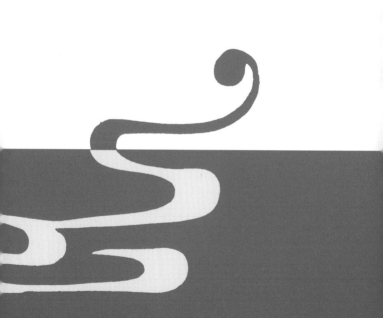

Cautiously, Confucius approached the old man and said to him, "I thought at first that you were some sort of spirit, but now I can see that you are a man of flesh and blood. Tell me, how in the world did you manage to survive that plunge into the river?"

"Oh that," answered the man. "That is simple. I merely entered the water at the center of its whirl. I let myself flow along with it, not trying to impose my will upon it, then I left when it whirled the opposite way. It is all completely natural to me."

"What do you mean by this?" asked Confucius. "How can this be natural to you?"

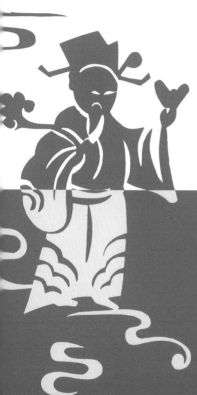

"Well," answered the man, already beginning to wander off again, "I grew up on dry land and so am at home upon it. At the same time, I also grew up by the river and so am at home in the water. I don't really know how I do these things, I just do them. Therefore my success is assured."

CHUANG TZU

We must respond differently to different situations; action should depend not only on subjective standards, but on the objective situation, to which we should adjust ourselves with the immediacy of the shadow adjusting itself to the moving body.

A.C. GRAHAM

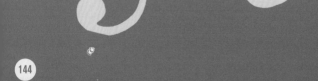

The highest good is like water.
Water gives life to the ten
thousand things and does not
strive. It flows in places men
reject and so is like the Tao.

LAO TZU

What is right in one case is not what is right in another; what is wrong in one case is not what is wrong in another.

HUAINANZI

Lieh Tzu was on his way to Chi but decided to turn back when he had gone halfway. He met his Master along the way who asked him why he had turned back.

"I was alarmed by something," he replied.

"What was it?" asked his Master.

Lieh explained that at every inn he was served first.

"Why was that such a problem?" asked his Master.

"When a man's inner integrity is not firm," said Lieh Tzu, "something oozes out of his body and becomes like an aura about him and presses on the hearts of others. It makes other men honor him more than his elders and gets him into difficulties."

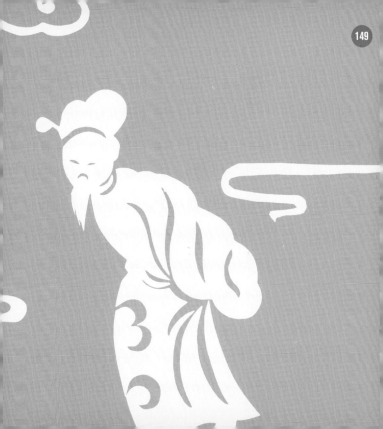

He then went on to describe that the motive of the innkeeper was to sell his wares and to make his profit. "If such a man as this values me so highly," he said, "think of how much worse it will be when the Great Lord finds out about me. He will appoint me to some office and insist that I fill it efficiently. This is what has alarmed me."

"An excellent way to look at it," said the Master. "But there is no way out of it. Even if you stay other men will lay responsibilities upon you."

LIEH TZU

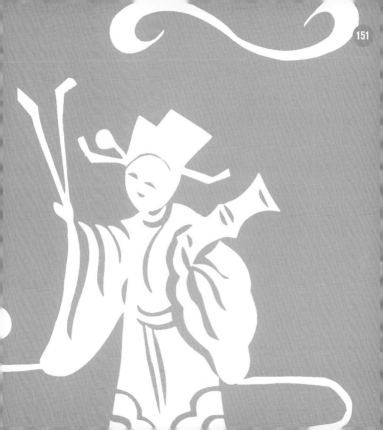

People follow the way of Earth;

Earth follows the way of Heaven;

Heaven follows the way of Tao;

Tao follows its own natural way.

LAO TZU

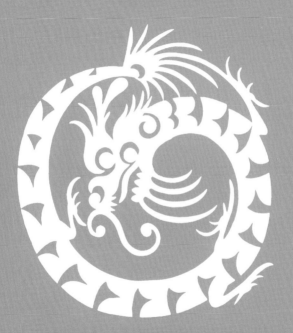

People in general bustle about here and there. The sage seems stupid and without "knowledge." When people dream they do not know that they are dreaming. In their dreamstate they may even pretend to interpret dreams. Only when they truly awaken do they begin to know that they have been dreaming. By and by will come the Great Awakening, and they shall find out that life itself is a great dream. All the while fools think that they are awake, and that they have knowledge. They go on making distinctions, they differentiate between princes and grooms. How stupid!

CHUANG TZU

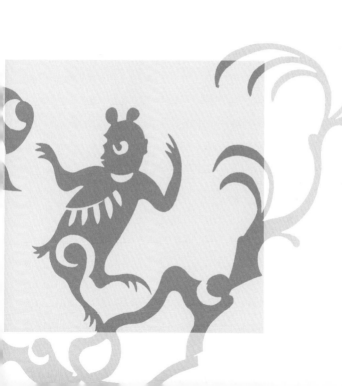

Not exalting the gifted prevents quarreling. Not valuing treasures prevents stealing. Not seeing desirable things prevents confusion of the heart.

LAO TZU

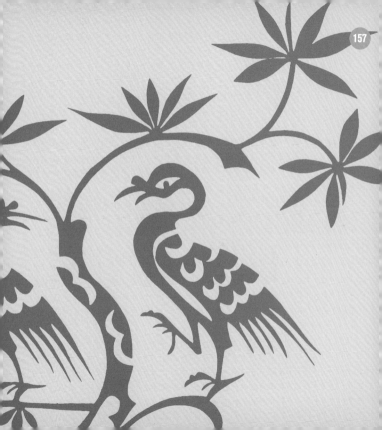

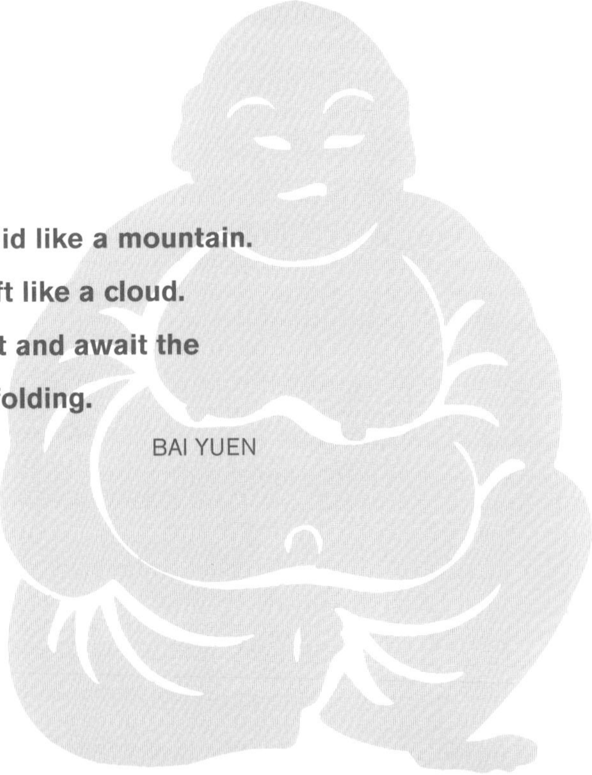

Solid like a mountain.

Soft like a cloud.

I sit and await the

unfolding.

BAI YUEN

Going with the flow means knowing just what the flow is in any given situation. This means attaining a deep level of sensitivity to the currents of each unfolding moment.

Lao-Tzu said:

"Those who attain the Way are weak in ambition but strong at work; their minds are open and their responses are fitting. Those weak in ambition are flexible and yielding, peaceful and quiet; they hide in nonacquisitiveness and pretend to be inexpert. Tranquil and untroubled, they act but they do miss the timing."

WEN TZU

Our culture is based on speed—everyone rushing to get ahead of the next guy, or perhaps just to keep up with him! Our brains are being trained to work faster and faster in order to keep up with the computers we have created, supposedly to make our work easier!

It is very difficult to hear that still, small voice from within when our brains are so filled with static from the world around us. We need to stop, slow down, and learn how to discern the inner flow of each moment as it unfolds from the one before it and then is enfolded by the one that follows.

Wu wei is about learning to conserve our energy and not spend it frivolously or in fear or confusion. Sometimes, rather than doing the wrong thing in a given situation, it is better to do nothing at all or to find some way around the situation rather than trying to batter our way through it.

John Blofeld tells us that:
"a Taoist conserves his
energy by easily according
with and adapting himself
to each situation."

It is in learning to adapt,
to flow with change, to
humble ourselves, that we
can save ourselves from
the stress and strain of
modern life.

The reason heaven and earth alone can last and endure is that they are tranquil; they give and do not seek to be repaid.

HO-SHANG KUNG

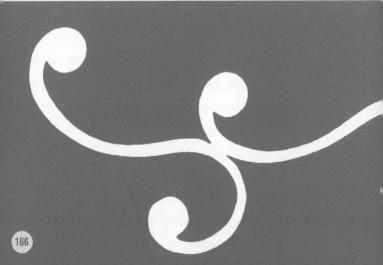

Follow the nature of things, without discriminating or separating them; thus no flaw or blame can reach you.

WANG PI

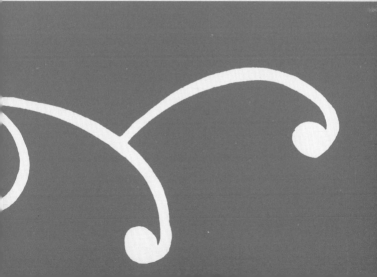

A Taoist conserves his energy by easily according with and adapting himself to each situation.

JOHN BLOFELD

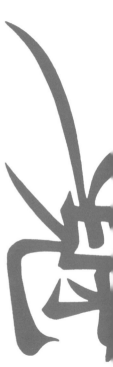

When people have a low cycle, they think of it in an emotional way and feel terrible. They want to die or kill themselves, they feel boring, unattractive and uninteresting, they don't realize that their low cycle can make them wise. Life is built up by each uninteresting moment, not just by excitement.

HUA CHING NI

Give and you will receive.
Be open-minded and soft-
hearted and friends will flock to
you. Be generous and humble
and you will be marked for
greatness. Do not try to attain
greatness and you will be
peaceful and happy.

For a human being to rediscover
his spontaneity, he must first
come to know the laws and
secrets of the universe, beginning
with those of his inner universe.

KRISTOFER SCHIPPER

To blame the Tao for not working while we are living in a polluted world is like tying down a unicorn from two directions and expecting it to run a thousand miles.

Place a monkey in a cage, and it is the same as a pig, not because it isn't clever and quick, but because it has no place to freely exercise its capabilities.

HUAINANZI

The sage practices nonaction.
She teaches by not speaking,
Achieves in all things while
undertaking nothing,
Creates but does not take credit,
Acts but does not depend,
Accomplishes much while not
claiming merit.
Because she claims no merit,
Her work will last forever.

LAO TZU

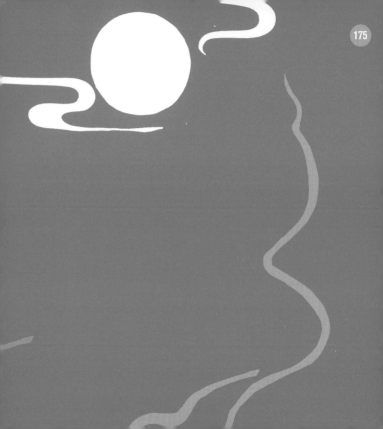

Slow down, become quiet, see with the inner eye, act from your true nature, stop trying, practice speaking without words, give without seeking reward and everything you seek will come to you.

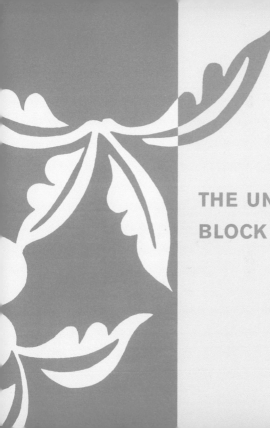

THE UNCARVED
BLOCK

The principle of the Uncarved Block, or *P'u*, is an essential element of Taoist thought. The story is told of the master carver who, after fasting and meditating for days to clear his inner vision, wanders out into the forest, looking at each tree and divining the inner shape.

In this way he is able to find just which tree inherently contains the shape of the carving he is seeking to create. Then, after taking the tree back to his studio, his only job is to remove all the layers of extraneous wood and reveal the inner sculpture and the shape he desires.

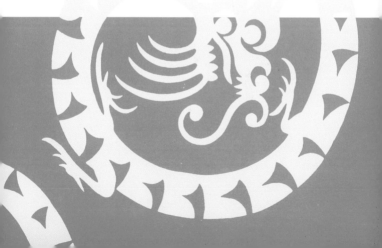

We too, as master carvers of our own lives, can reshape and reform our own experience of the world. Our culture, our society, our environment, our family, and our own personal experiences have covered us in layer upon layer of unnatural material which obscures our essential nature.

It is in removing these layers and uncovering the natural form within that we can find our true selves. In this way we each exist as an Uncarved Block, ready to free the inner sculpture that exists under all the layers of artificiality where our own true nature resides.

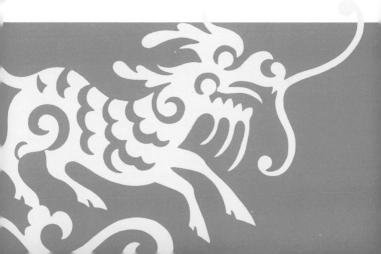

Fame or life: which is more desired?
Life or goods: which is greater?
Gain or loss: which is more harmful?
Those who are attached will suffer;
Those who hoard will suffer losses;
Those who know when they have
enough will not be disgraced;
Those who know how to stop will
not be harmed;
They will go on forever.

LAO TZU

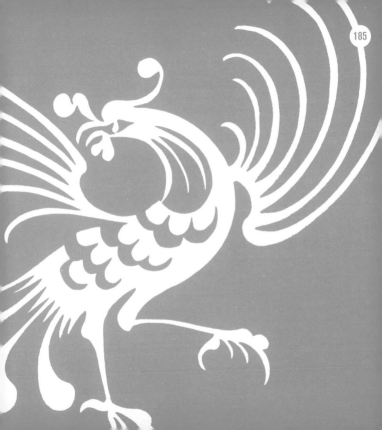

"Rabbit's very clever," said Pooh thoughtfully.

"Yes," said Piglet, "Rabbit's clever."

"And he has a brain."

"Yes," said Piglet, "Rabbit has a brain."

There was a long silence.

"I suppose," said Pooh, "that's why he never understands anything."

A.A. MILNE, *WINNIE THE POOH*

The joy for the Taoist is that things have no use, and the future is not important.

ALAN WATTS

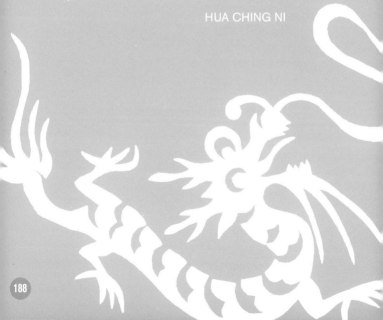

The principles treasured by the Taoist
are simplicity, equilibrium, harmony,
and quietude.

HUA CHING NI

While on the Path
of Tao everything
unfolds naturally
and there is
nothing left to do.

Thirty spokes share one hub;
It is the empty space within that
makes it useful.
Clay is shaped into a vessel;
It is the empty space that
makes it useful.
Cut out doors and windows
And it is the empty spaces
created that makes them useful.
Profit comes for what is there;
Usefulness by what is not there.

LAO TZU

A certain carpenter was traveling with his helper. They came to a town where a giant oak tree filled the square. It was huge, with many limbs traveling far out over the square. It was large enough to shade a hundred oxen and its shade covered the entire square. The helper was amazed at the possibility of lumber contained in this one tree but the carpenter passed it by with a mere glance. When his helper asked him why he had passed up such a magnificent specimen the carpenter replied that he could see at one glance that the great oak's branches were useless to him.

"They are so hard," he said, "that were I to take my axe to them it would split it. The wood is so heavy that a boat made of it would sink. The branches themselves are so gnarled and twisted they cannot be made into planks. If I tried to fashion house beams with it, it would collapse. If I made a coffin from it you would not be able to fit someone inside. Altogether it is a completely useless tree. And that is the secret of its long life."

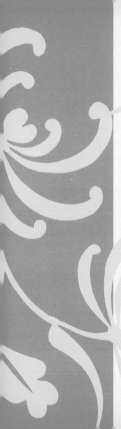

The trees on the mountain can
be used to build and so are cut
down.
When fat is added to the fire it
consumes itself.
Cinnamon can be eaten and so
is harvested.
The lacquer tree can be used
and so is slashed.
Everyone knows the usefulness
of the useful.
But no one knows the
usefulness of the useless!

CHUANG TZU

To overdo, to emphasize productivity, to oversharpen the blade is to invite disaster. When will the world acknowledge the worth of the mundane, the value of the ordinary, the utter precariousness of the commonplace?

In a back lane a sage quietly lived a simple
life, having just enough food to keep himself
alive. Poor and miserable though he might
seem, yet he felt happy and held himself
in high esteem.

WONG TAI SIN

The realized person unites her nature with that of Tao. She is full yet to others seems empty. She abides in the Oneness, that is all she knows. She is able to govern herself inwardly and does not notice what is external.

HUAINANZI

Sages learn how
to return their
own nature to the
true Nature of Tao
and let their mind
wander freely in
the infinite.

A simple, plain, and
natural life is essential
spiritual completeness.

HUA CHING NI

The emptiness between
heaven and earth
is like a bellows.
It is empty but does not
lose its form.
It can be moved but it
stretches even further.
Words do not count,
Maintain the center.

LAO TZU

Stop filling when the vessel is full.
A knife sharpened too often will
not retain its edge.
If gold and jade fill your home it
will be impossible to defend.
Arrogant wealth and rank will
bring its own punishment.
Withdraw after good deeds,
This is the Way of Tao.

LAO TZU

There was once a highly educated and somewhat arrogant student of the Way who went to visit the renowned master so that the sage could show him a few things he might not yet know.

"Please sit down and join me in some tea, honorable sir," offered the old man.

They sat and, while the student boasted about his education and recounted his many accomplishments, the old master began to fill his guest's tea cup.

As the student rambled on and on so too did the old master keep pouring tea into his cup until the hot tea overflowed across the table and poured onto the student's lap.

"What are you doing, you old dolt?" he shrieked, leaping from his chair. "You are spilling tea everywhere. Can't you see that my cup is already full?"

The sage calmly stopped pouring tea and looked at him. "Your mind, sir, is much like this tea cup. I'm afraid it is already too full for me to be able to fit anything else into. Else it will surely run over and spill everywhere."

So too must we be willing to empty our minds and hearts of preconceived notions of knowledge and ideas of importance and accomplishment.

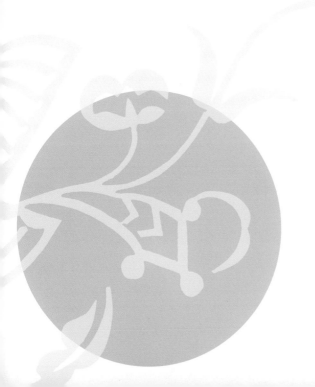

We must empty
ourselves
before we are
fit to receive.

In the world of knowledge,
Every day something new
is added.
In pursuit of the Tao, every
day something is let go.

LAO TZU

True understanding
follows when one
learns how useful it
is to be useless.

After studying with his master for many years the ancient sage Lieh Tzu decided that, in truth, he had never really learned anything. So he went home and for three years did not leave his house.

He cooked meals for his wife,

Served food to his pigs as though

they were human,

Treated all things as equally as

his kin,

From carved jade he returned to

the unhewn block,

Till his single shape stood forth,

detached from all things.

He was free of tangles

Once and for all, to the end

of his life.

LIEH TZU

The Tao does not judge, it does not punish, it does not condemn. We do that ourselves. And as we judge, so too can we forgive—ourselves and others who have wronged us through their own mistaken sense of reality.

Through forgiveness, through trust, through taking chances with ourselves and others, and through returning to our "original nature"—our own sweet simple and natural self, our own "uncarved block"—we can begin the journey that leads back to its beginning, to our original nature, or Tao.

You must return to your natural self, to *p'u*. You must discard morality and ambition, for if you keep those you will never be capable of compassion, moderation and humility. When you discard some of your wishes, you will have them all.

HUA CHING NI

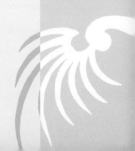

In eating, it is best not to fill up;

In thinking, it is best not to overdo.

KUAN TZU

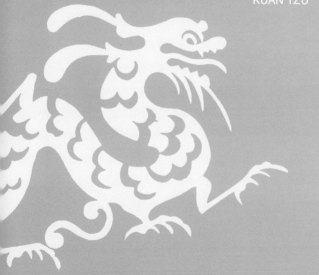

Clubfoot-Hunchback-No-Lips came to see Duke Ling. Duke Ling who, after speaking with him, became so delighted with him that when he saw normal people, it seemed to him that their legs looked thin and spindly.

Jug-Neck-Goiter came to see the Duke of Chi. He so impressed the Duke that when he saw normal people he thought their necks looked thin and scraggy.

When one's personal integrity shines forth one's outward appearance will be forgotten. By not forgetting what should be forgotten and forgetting what should not be forgotten—that is called true forgetfulness!

CHUANG TZU

True spiritual cultivation
begins with the premise
that you already have a
pure spirit and only need
to clear any obfuscations.

DENG MING DAO

Those who know when they have enough are the wealthiest in the world.

Become simple, become natural.
Delve into the core of your being
And let your true self free!

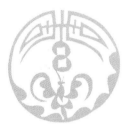

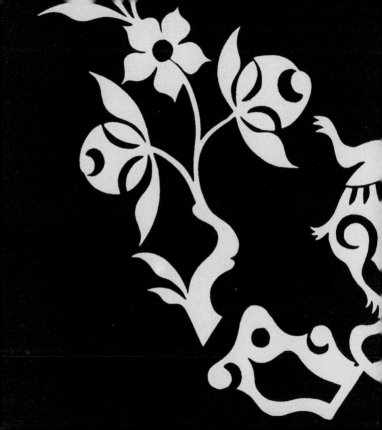

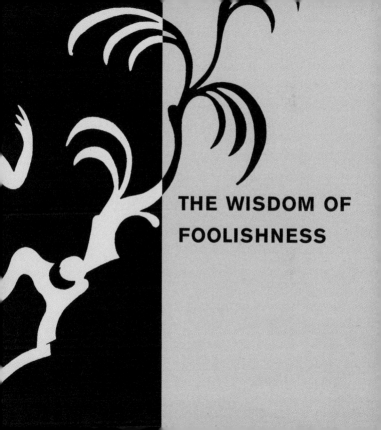

THE WISDOM OF
FOOLISHNESS

One of the truly unique aspects of the Path of Tao is the Wisdom of Foolishness, sometimes called Crazy Wisdom.

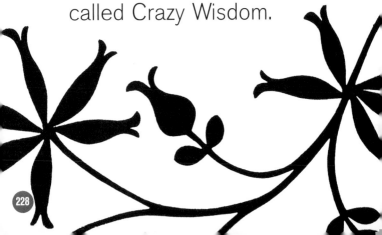

The use of paradox, inversion, wordplay, metaphor, and humor mark it as a special form of teaching. Many of what we might consider Zen stories have their origin in Taoism. Indeed the origins of Zen come from the Tao.

Buddhism entered China around 600 C.E. It was mixed with the native Path of Tao and became a form of Buddhism called Chan, which took many aspects of Taoism—nonreliance on scriptures and priests, the immediacy of being in the moment, the importance of direct experience and the use of meditation. This new form of Buddhism then moved to Japan, where it was taken up by the Samurai class who laid a thick layer of bushido philosophy over it and where it became what we know today as Zen.

But the use of outrageous stories of seemingly foolish and oftentimes outright bizarre teachers and their interactions with their students and their community all comes from the tradition of Taoism.

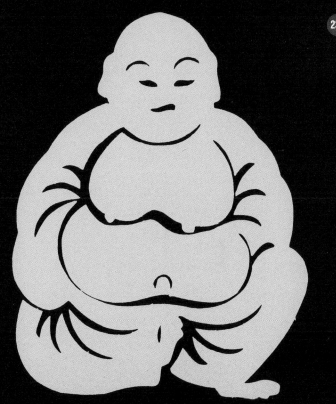

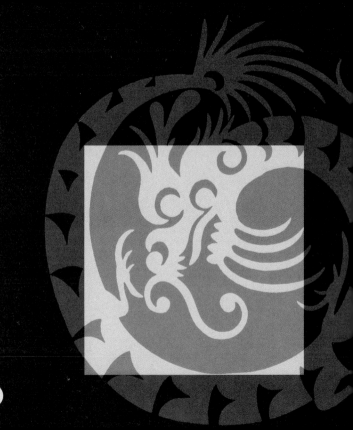

It is through playful stories that we can see the inner workings of the mind of the sage, who is beyond the strictures of society and the so-called morality of the times. A morality that is, in reality, a form of social and cultural control and has nothing to do with real spirituality.

When the great Tao is abandoned,

benevolence and morality arise.

When wisdom and intelligence arise,

There comes a great falseness.

When the family is not united,

Filial piety and kindness arise.

When the country is full of confusion

and disorder,

Then loyal court ministers appear.

LAO TZU

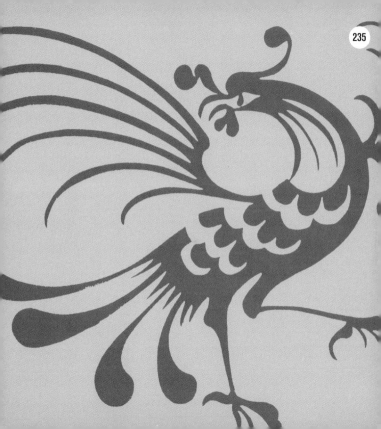

The Realized (Authentic) Person is free, like the wind and water; living their life unattached to appearances and form, understanding the true essence of all things and all beings.

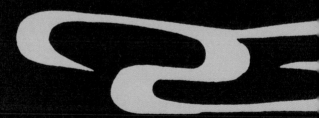

Where can I find a man
who has forgotten
words? I would like to
have a word with him.

CHUANG TZU

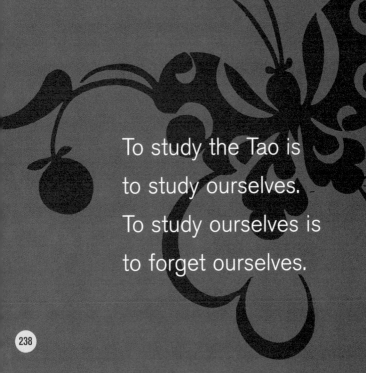

To study the Tao is
to study ourselves.
To study ourselves is
to forget ourselves.

Taoists and Zen masters learn to ride the currents and surrender to the flow. They become friends with insecurity, making doubt their guide and each moment their god.

WES NISKER

Right is not right; so is not so. If right were really right, it would differ so from not right that there would be no need for argument. If so were really so, it would differ so clearly from not so that there would be no need for argument. Forget the years; forget distinctions. Leap into the boundless and make it your home!

CHUANG TZU

The student came up to the master. "This thing you call Tao," he said, throwing wide his arms. "Where does it exist?"

The master stood for a moment then pointed to a steaming pile of ox manure. "It is there," he said.

Once, a great Lord sent his envoys to the old master who sat on his backside on the riverbank, lazily fishing. They had come to invite him to come back to the court with them where he would be installed as a Royal Sage. Though to look at him, the old man certainly did not look much like a sage, as he sat idly scratching himself in the midday sun.

After the royal envoys had told him of their mission the old man looked at them for a long moment. The envoys were a little puzzled. They had expected the old man to jump at the chance for a life of ease and comfort in the capital. He certainly didn't look like he was doing too well out here in the countryside.

Finally the old man asked, "Is it true that you have an ancient tortoise shell up there at the capital?" That was true. The tortoise shell was used for divination and was said to be over three thousand years old. After they had answered yes, the old man looked at them for another long moment.

"Do you suppose," he asked, "that if the tortoise had been given the choice to be killed in order to give up its shell to be used by the court or be left alone to drag its tail through the mud, which would it have chosen?"

The envoys, a bit shaken by this strange question, answered that, of course, if given the choice, the tortoise would have chosen to be left alone to "drag its tail through the mud."

"Well then," said the old man, turning his mud-stained backside to them. "Go away and leave me to drag mine through the mud!"

Opposites depend on each other for existence and have no independent meaning. The Taoist holy fools stand right in the middle of paradox, where all dualities converge.

WES NISKER

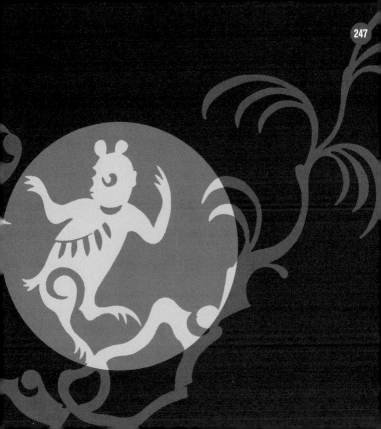

Give up learning and put an end to your troubles.

LAO TZU

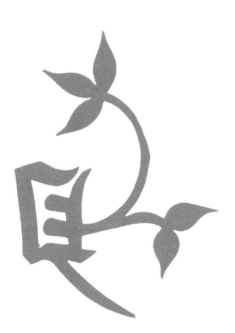

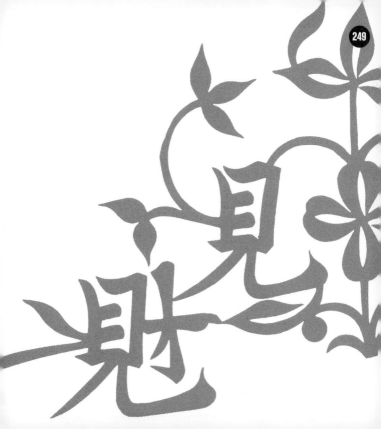

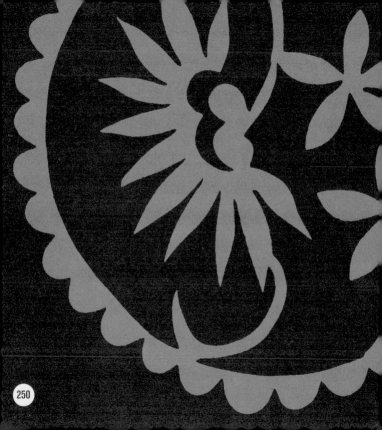

Give up sagehood,
renounce wisdom
And the people will
benefit a hundredfold.

LAO TZU

Put an end to wisdom that leaves tracks and reason that deceives, and people will benefit greatly.

WANG CHEN

The Realized Person of ancient
times slept without dreaming
and woke without fear.
Their food was simple and
their breathing was deep.

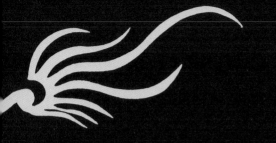

When you try to understand everything, you will not understand anything. The best way is to understand yourself, and then you will understand everything.

SHUNRU SUZUKI

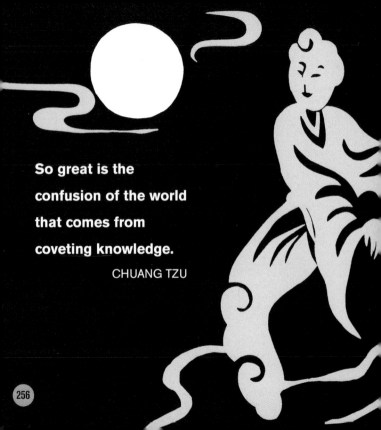

So great is the
confusion of the world
that comes from
coveting knowledge.

CHUANG TZU

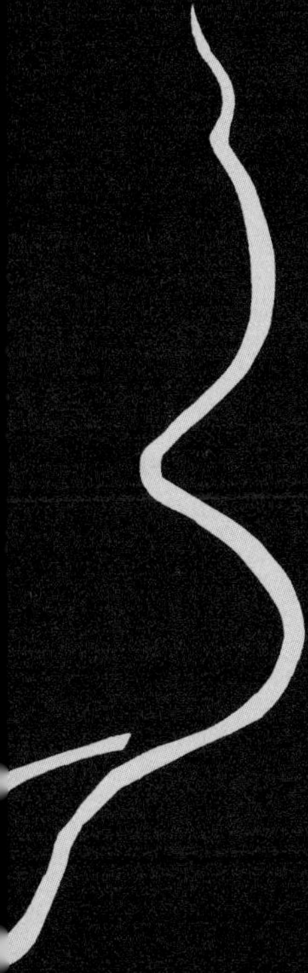

A truly wise person
is not aware of
her wisdom,
therefore she is wise.
A truly foolish person
tries to be wise,
And therefore is not.

The sage dwells on what
is profound and deep
And not on what is
only surface.
They dwell in what is
eternal and not what
is transient.
They prefer the fruit
over the flower.

**If we listen with a quiet mind
and do not let our ideas distract
us, we will understand others
even before words are spoken.**

EVA WONG

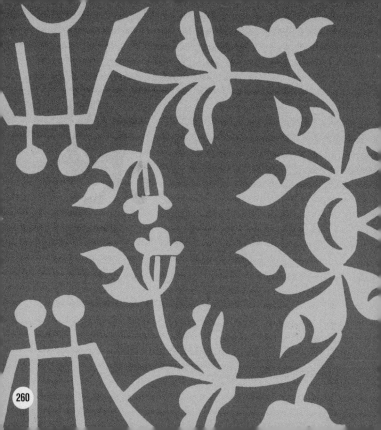

When the superior person hears of the Tao
He diligently studies it.
When the inferior person hears of the Tao
Sometimes she remembers it, sometimes not.
When the foolish student hears of the Tao
They laugh at it.
If they did not laugh at it,
It would not be the Tao.

LAO TZU

There are teachers everywhere, in all kinds of places. Lao Tzu, Chuang Tzu, and Lieh Tzu are just three of the vast numbers of Taoist teachers and sages who have shared their wisdom with us over the centuries. But many masters of Tao are experts in invisibility. They don't proclaim themselves to the world as enlightened beings.

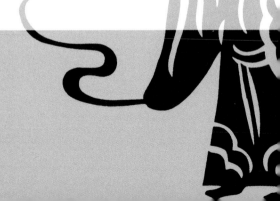

They don't run huge glossy ads in New Age magazines. They are not even recognizable at first glance.

They could be living next door to you and you'd never know it until you learned to see with the eye of the heart (an old way of saying with the eye of discriminating consciousness).

Lao Tzu said that a good man is the teacher of a not good man. And the not good man is the good man's responsibility. He then goes further to say that if the teacher is not respected and the student is not cared for, although there may be great

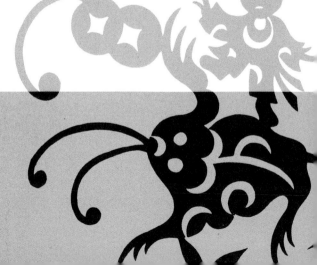

knowledge there will be great confusion. This is called the Deep Mystery.

Even more mysterious is the often confusing tale of the "holy fools" or what is also called in the Path of Tao, "The Wisdom of Foolishness."

The Tao is hidden by partial understanding. The true meaning of words is hidden by flowery rhetoric.

CHUANG TZU

She who knows she is a fool
is therefore not a fool. He
who knows he is confused
is not so confused.

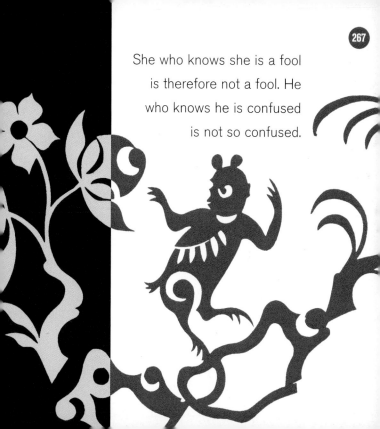

Take the "s" out of cosmic and enjoy what's left.

CHUNGLIANG AL HUANG

Angels fly because they

take themselves so lightly.

G.K. CHESTERTON

It is difficult to be muddleheaded, and difficult to be intelligent. It is even more difficult to graduate from intelligence into muddleheadedness.

CHEN PAN-CH'AO

The torch of doubt and chaos, this is what the sage steers by.

CHUANG TZU

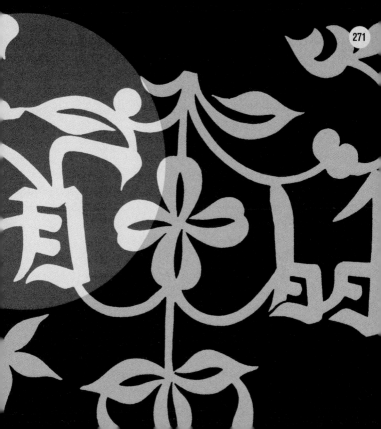

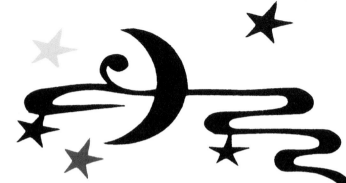

A student asked the master, "I do not ask you anything about pointing, what is the moon?"

The master asked back, "Who is not asking about pointing?"

Another student asked, "I do not ask you about the moon, what is pointing?"

The master replied, "The moon."

The student then said, "I asked about pointing, why did you speak of the moon?"

The master answered, Because you asked about pointing."

True wisdom is like ripe fruit.

When one tries to hold it too hard

It flies out of your grasp

And lands in the mud!

Don't limit your vision only
to yourself; benefit others
with your good humor.

CHUNGLIANG AL HUANG

I cannot tell if what the world considers "happiness" is happiness or not. All I know is that when I consider the way they go about attaining it, I see them carried away headlong, grim and obsessive, in the general onrush of the human herd, unable to stop themselves or to change their direction. All the while they claim to be just on the point of attaining happiness. My opinion is that you never find happiness until you stop looking for it.

CHUANG TZU

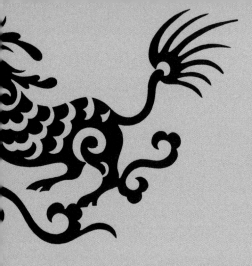

The answers to all our questions are hidden everywhere, just outside our line of sight—that is, until we open our eyes a little wider and begin looking around us instead of just straight ahead. They jump out at us from everywhere, displaying themselves in all their stunning simplicity.

The student came to the master and said, "Please help me to quiet my mind."

The master answered, "Bring me your mind and I promise I will help you."

The student stood there for a moment and then said, "But Master, I cannot seem to find it."

"Ah," replied the master, "then I quieted it."

Nature, while not always beneficent, contains its own inherent order. So do we, as natural beings, contain our own inherent order.

Confusion comes from trying to deviate from that order.

The essential nature of water is clear, but dirt mixed in it will obscure it. The essential nature of people is peaceful, but too many desires will damage it. The sage is one who can leave the world of things and return to the original self.

The master sat, silently, with closed eyes. Her student came up to and stood before her. After a few moments the master opened her eyes and, with her finger, drew a circle on the ground before her. In the circle she wrote the word *water*. Then she looked up at the student who looked back, saying nothing.

The master asked the student, "What is your name?" The student replied, "Spiritual Pervasion." The master held up a lantern. "Then please enter this lantern." The student turned away. "I am already inside it," he said. The master shook his head and said, "Then there is no hope for you."

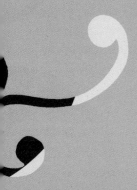

A path is formed by walking on it. A thing has a name because of its being called something. Why is it like this? Because it is! Why is it not like that? Because it is not! Everything has its own nature and function.

CHUANG TZU

A student once asked Hsiang Yen, "What is Tao?"

Hsiang Yen replied, "A dragon hums inside a withered log."

Other people have more than enough

But I alone seem to have lost everything.

I am foolish!

Other people are clear

While I alone am confused.

Other people are clever

While I am stupid.

I feel lost at sea,

Tossed about on the winds of a storm.

Everyone else has things to do

While I am dull and stupid.

I am different from the others.

I am nourished by the Great Mother.

LAO TZU

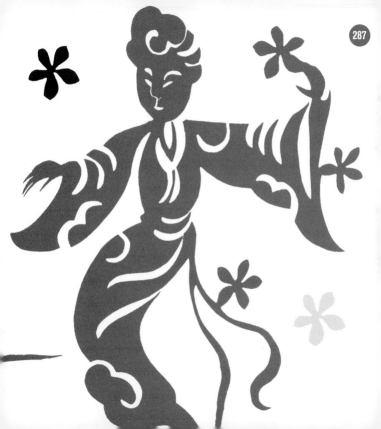

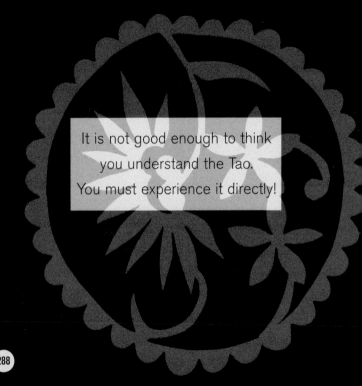

It is not good enough to think
you understand the Tao.
You must experience it directly!

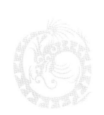

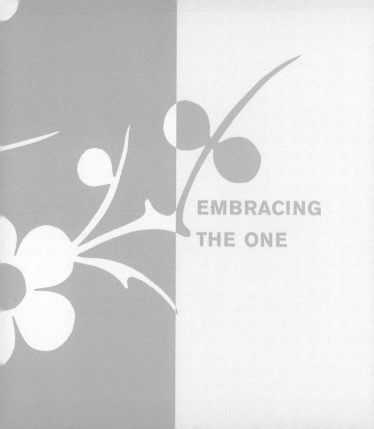

EMBRACING
THE ONE

Embracing the One, sometimes called Returning to the Source, is the phrase used on the Path of Tao for that deeply connective and mystical place found in Taoist meditation practices. Taoist meditation practice is a bit different from many other forms of meditation or contemplation. This is primarily due to the emphasis on energy work. There is, of course, the basic practice of quieting the mind. But we also use the mind to guide *chi* or primal energy throughout the body—toning, healing, detoxifying, and strengthening organs, muscles, and lymph glands; bringing the whole system into harmony.

In Chinese it is called *ching jing wu wei,* sitting still and doing nothing. To an outside observer we may look as though we are simply sitting or standing quietly, but the reality is that on the inside, we may be running energy or *chi* throughout our body or through the microcosmic orbit (usually up the back and down the front). Or we may be cooking up healing elixirs in the lower *dan tien* (lower abdomen). It is here, in what the ancient Taoists called the cauldron or "the field of medicine," that we can mix internal energies and create healing *chi* that can then move throughout our body.

Here great forces are at work, rerouting and reshaping streams of energy and light, changing the very internal being of the meditator. This is all part of the process or journey back to our original divine state, our own experience of Tao.

It is in slowing down, stopping the outward senses, and looking deeply within that we can find our way on the Great Way, and in that journey come to experience ourselves as part of the Source of all Life.

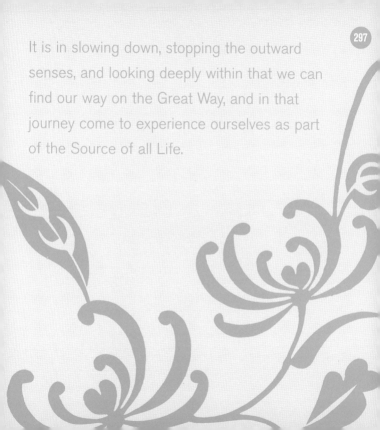

Returning to the source is a figurative term for the unutterably blissful experience of becoming aware with all one's being of perfect identity with all that is, has been, or ever could be.

JOHN BLOFELD

Best be still, best be empty.

In stillness and emptiness we find where to

abide; Talking and giving, we lose the place.

LIEH TZU

By calming the mind,
by watching the
breath, by clearing
the emotions, by
allowing each
moment to pass
unobstructed we can
enter the vast flow
of the Eternal Tao.

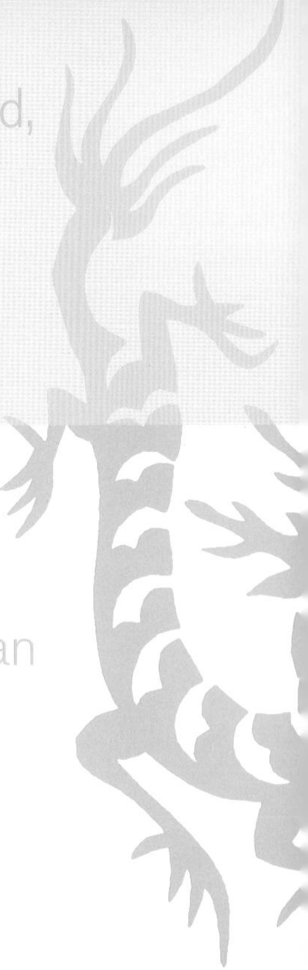

Who can be still while the
muddy water settles?
Who can remain still until
the time comes for action?

LAO TZU

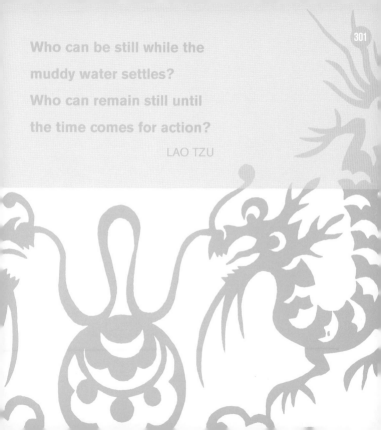

It is impossible to attain
inner stillness without first
attaining outer stillness.

Practice to become empty,
Let your mind become tranquil.
Let each moment go by on its own,
While you silently observe.
This is called Returning to the Source.

The real point of sitting still and doing nothing is to empty the mind entirely of all conceptual thought, and let the spirit abide in emptiness, silence, and stillness.

DANIEL REID

Too few devote even one
second to entering deeply
the great current of life
hidden within ourselves.

MANTAK CHIA

Breathing deeply and slowly, from the belly, we allow our thoughts, feelings, and emotions to settle like water that has been mixed with silt. As the silt settles to the bottom the water becomes clear and pure.

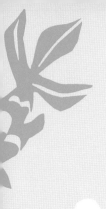

Count your breaths, slowly, from one to ten, concentrating fully on each count. Then once you reach ten, go back and start over again.

While sitting one must always keep the heart quiet and the power concentrated. How can the heart be made quiet? By breathing.

LU TZU

Although the breath that flows in and out through the nose is not the true breath, the flowing in and out of the true breath is connected with it.

LU TZU

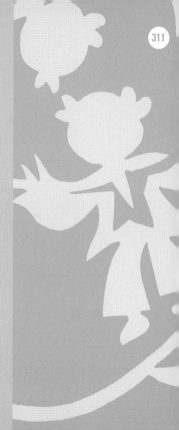

Let meditation assist
your life, do not use
it to spin a cocoon
around your life.

HUA CHING NI

To be like a heap of
clods or a pile of dust
is perverse, even
though it is Doing
Nothing.

LIEH TZU

Taoist meditation, just like Taoist philosophy, requires a flexible attitude. You have to be careful not to hold yourself too stiffly. As Hua Ching Ni, a contemporary Taoist master says, "If your attitude towards meditation is too tight and you sit solemnly

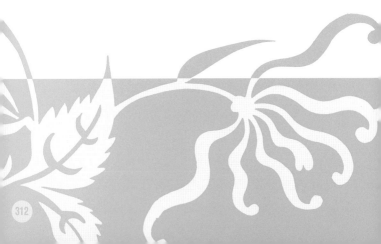

and stiffly, you will increase this overly serious and unpleasant aspect of your practice and this will become the fruit you bear. If, on the other hand, you sit with genuine joy, the world sings to you; the pores and cells of the breeze dance for you."

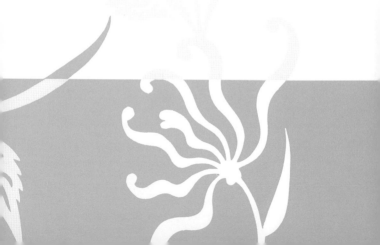

Remember to keep an attitude of openness, receptivity, joy, and engaged relaxation as you sit. Allow yourself to be carried on the currents of energy and spirit and let yourself discover the hidden depths of your soul.

Lu Dong Bin, one of the famous Taoist Immortals described meditation:

"As for the stages experienced through the exercise of quiescence, first there is dullness, oblivion, and random thought; then there is lightness and freshness; later it is like being inside curtains of gold mesh; finally it is like returning to life from death, a clear breeze under the bright moon coming and going, the scenery unobstructed."

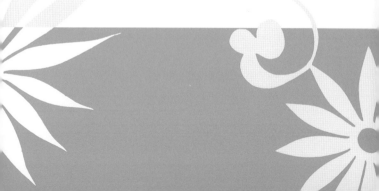

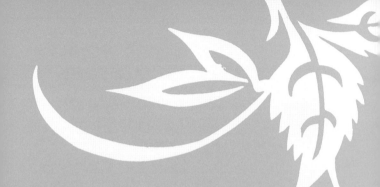

If nothing within you stays rigid,

Outward things will disclose

themselves.

Moving, be like water.

Still, be like a mirror.

Respond like an echo.

KUAN YIN

Without going out your door,

You can know the whole world.

Without looking through your window,

You can see the Tao of Heaven.

LAO TZU

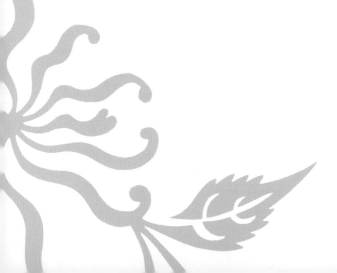

Meditation is not possible for the unimaginative, the stupid, or the dogmatic. Meditation requires a plunging into the creative, a suspension of the everyday logical mind that stands in the way of our efforts. It is only when we go behind this petty, rationalistic mind that extraordinary experiences become possible.

DENG MING DAO

While Western science had to wait until the development of equipment sufficiently sensitive to observe, measure, and record light waves, electric pulses, and atomic particles, Taoists simply "sat still and did nothing" long enough to awaken their own inner reflections of the universe.

DANIEL REID

Most of what we know today as the meridian system, which is used in Traditional Chinese Medicine and *chi kung*, was mapped by those "inner astronauts", the ancient Taoists, who, while sitting in deep meditation, were able to track how and where energy moved in their bodies.

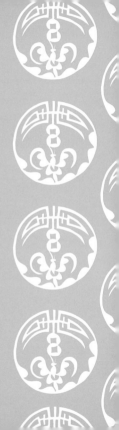

"*Qi* follows *yi*." *Chi* follows the mind. Use your conscious intent to send healing energy or light to the parts of your body that are in pain, diseased, or feeling toxic.

Relaxation does not mean loss of control. Relaxing your body doesn't mean letting it go limp. It means dispelling all tension, and allowing the inherent energy of your body to flow freely. In this sense, relaxation releases energy.

DENG MING DAO

Correct relaxation is not collapse. It is an energetic, dynamic type of relaxation in which your muscles, tendons, organs, and nervous system get a chance to refresh and re-energize themselves.

Sitting quietly, on a cushion or edge of chair, eyes closed or half closed. Relaxing our shoulders, we begin to breathe deeply and slowly, from the belly, placing the tip of our tongue on our upper palate. Deep in our lower *dan tien*, our "field of elixir," we feel a golden ball expanding and contracting with each inhale and each exhale. We feel it expanding into our whole abdomen, filling us with golden healing light.

As we continue to breathe we inhale fresh *chi* or primal energy, from the atmosphere surrounding us. We feel it move into our nose and down our throat and into our lungs. Using our mind we breathe it all the way into our lower abdomen, our *dan tien*. Then, on each exhale, we breathe out all toxins, stress, disease, and negative emotions like a thin black cloud. In and out, the exchange of healing *chi* and toxic or "dirty" *chi*, goes on, until we feel ourselves full of healthy, vibrant *chi* and clear of any stresses, tension or toxins—be they mental, emotional or physical.

Relaxing our face into a small smile we relax slowly into our being and allow ourselves to be breathed!

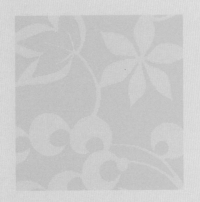

Hold the body and spirit as one.

Can you avoid their separation?

Concentrating your *chi* and

becoming pliant,

Can you become like a

newborn baby?

Clearing your mind and

contemplating the profound,

Can you remain unflawed?

LAO TZU

In understanding all things
Can you remain apart from them?
Can you bear the fruit without
taking possession of it?
Can you do the work without
taking the credit?
Can you act without taking control?
Can you lead without dominating?
Can speak without speaking?
Can you sit without moving?

This is called the profound and
secret virtue.

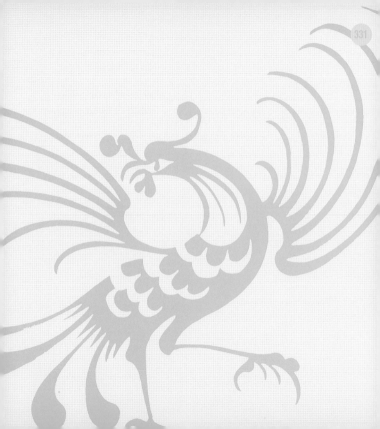

What is this state of spiritual receptivity? It means that when you are completely relaxed and empty of any desire, you will become receptive to inspiration.

KE YUN LU

Make your mind and your thoughts like a mirror, reflecting all that comes in view without holding on to any of it.

Those who are unable to attain the Tao are those whose minds are not clear and who are still slaves of their emotions.

T'AI SHANG CH'ING-CHING CHING

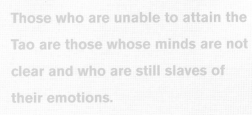

Meditation is not
mystical or magical.
Meditation is who
you are when you are
not thinking about
who you are!

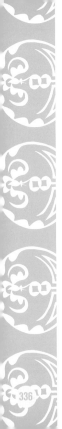

The highest achievement as a Taoist
is the refinement of one's spirit into
an irresistible precious sword which
can cut through all mental obstacles
and impediments.

HUA CHING NI

Use energy to help
energy; do not always
rely on the mind.

HUA CHING NI

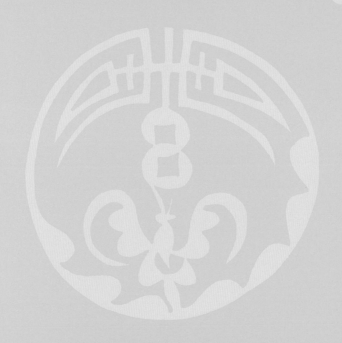

The trick, of meditation, is to be able to maintain some semblance of a meditative state even in the midst of your daily activities. It is one thing to be able to still the mind and quiet the heart while breathing deeply and sitting on one's own meditation cushion.

It is quite another to be able to maintain that sense of calmness and quietude when confronted by the stresses and fears which we encounter when we leave our cushion.

It is crucial that we learn how to take the insights and self-knowledge we gain in meditation and carry that over into the rest of our life. It can be as simple as keeping your breath slow and deep, and from the belly, at all times, especially when you feel tense or stressed.

Oftentimes, the things we learn about ourselves in deep meditation are not always pleasant. Your own monkey mind will try and fight you all the way, coming up with ever more thoughts that are connected to other thoughts that are connected to yet more thoughts and so on and on.

When meditating, do not allow the thoughts to take over and also not to try so desperately not to think. Just let each thought emerge, like taking a breath, and then let it go, like exhaling. Eventually they will slow down of their own accord and you can then dwell in the land of no-thought.

Stay comprehensively alert in the immediate present, and suddenly an awakening will open up an experience in the midst of it all that is millions of times better than that of quiet sitting.

HUANG YUAN-CH'I

When we are quiet, still, calm, and empty, it is much easier to experience true spiritual wisdom. When we are stressed, moving too quickly, angry or fearful, it is so much harder to hold to the center. It is then that we make mistakes, cause accidents, create regrets, and lose our place.

When your brows are knitted because of worry, not only is your body knitted, but your internal organs are also tightened into knots.

KE YUN LU

Taoists believe that we are born with a precious jewel in our heart, a drop of spirit which unites us with the Eternal Tao. It is within us yet it is not ours alone, but

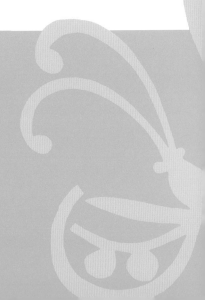

held in common with all other human beings. When we nurture and refine that jewel through spiritual practice we can become what the ancients called Immortals.

Close your mouth.

Shut the door of desire

And you will live your life with no harm.

Stop acting and reacting

And you will have no problems.

Use the light to return to the Light.

Then you can die yet be ever living.

LAO TZU

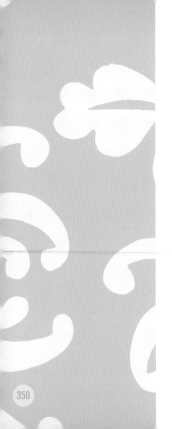

According to spiritual nature, we are the products of our environment and we are here to fulfill one great purpose; to use the body as a laboratory to do the work of self-refinement, which is also called internal alchemy.

HUA CHING NI

When we genuinely feel a loving kindness toward nature and men, we are already in a natural state of relaxation. We will be free and easy. That is when enlightenment dawns.

KE YUN LU

Returning is the direction of the Tao.

Yielding is the way of the Tao.

All things under heaven are born of being;

being is born of nonbeing.

LAO TZU

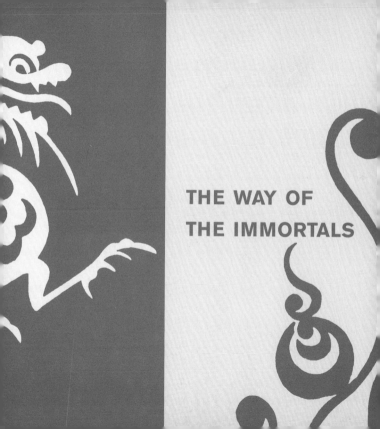

THE WAY OF
THE IMMORTALS

Often, on the Path of Tao we come across the term Immortal. This is usually taken to mean someone who has reached a level of spiritual attainment where they are said to have Entered the Tao. This is someone who has consciously reconnected themselves to their divine origin, the Tao itself. They are now free from the laws of time and the material world. They can come and go as they wish, leaving their bodies to travel on the spiritual planes. Their spiritual understanding is complete and they can become teachers, guides, and helpers to us all. In Buddhist terms, they have reached enlightenment.

When we use the term Immortal, it is not in the Western concept of someone who lives forever. Their spiritual self is immortal but they do leave their body when it is time. Indeed, they are not attached to their body, although they treat it as a holy temple. There are many famous immortals such as Lu Dong Bin, Chen Duan, Ko Hong but many of the immortals of history are nameless, humble people who have persevered in their self-cultivation until they have reached such a level of experience and understanding that their spiritual selves live on long after their physical bodies.

The ancient achieved ones

Were masters at penetrating the subtle and

profound Tao.

They were so deep that we cannot describe them.

They were cautious, like someone fording a

frozen river.

They were vigilant, like someone who is

surrounded by enemies.

They were courteous, like dignified guests.

They were ephemeral, like melting ice.

They were simple, like the uncarved block.

They were open and wide, like a valley.

They were deep, like swirling water.

LAO TZU

Become simple, become humble, become childlike, become open, become fearless, become empty, become whole. This is the Way of the Immortals!

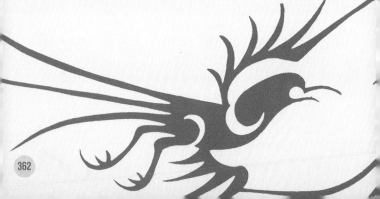

The Abbot of Loukuantai, a venerable and delightful old man, said to me: "The world thinks that it is going forward and that we Taoists are going backward, but really it is just the opposite; we are going forward and they are going backward."

JOSEPH NEEDHAM

Simple people who seek eternal life in the courts of heaven or as transmogrified flesh-and-blood immortals, philosophers who acquire the wisdom of acceptance in the manner of Lao-tzu, adepts of the yogic alchemy and mystics who pursue the exalted goal known as the return to the Source, one and all describe attainment with the words *ch'eng hsien*—becoming an immortal.

JOHN BLOFELD

The Way of the Immortals is the way of self-cultivation. By using your own innate talents plant the seeds of enlightenment within yourself and then cultivate them carefully as they grow.

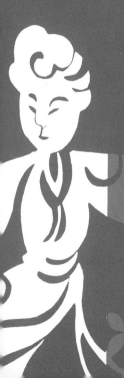

The deep truth cannot be learned from books alone but as a direct subtle revelation in your own sagely mind.

HUA CHING NI

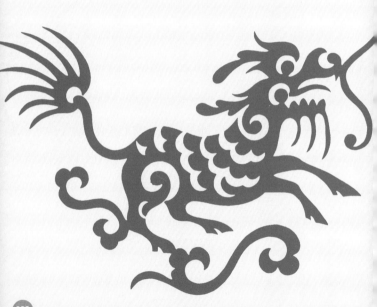

Entering the
Shadowy Portal,
they pass beyond
the world of dust
into the realm
of immortals.

Sojourning in the Ta-Yu Mountains,

Who converses with the white crane

That comes flying?

How many times have the mountain people

Seen the winter plum-flowers blossoming?

Spring comes and goes,

Deep in fallen flowers and streams.

People are not aware

Of the many Immortals around them.

LU DONG BIN

In not showing off
She is seen by everyone.
In not being self-satisfied,
She is prominent.
In not being too aggressive
She accomplishes all her tasks.
In not boasting
She is admired by all.
Because she does not contend
No one contends with her.
The ancients said:
To yield is to become whole.

LAO TZU

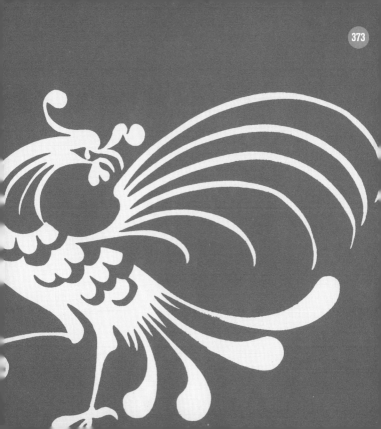

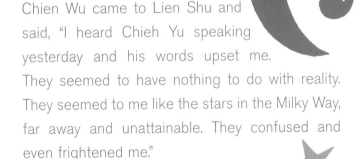

Chien Wu came to Lien Shu and said, "I heard Chieh Yu speaking yesterday and his words upset me. They seemed to have nothing to do with reality. They seemed to me like the stars in the Milky Way, far away and unattainable. They confused and even frightened me."

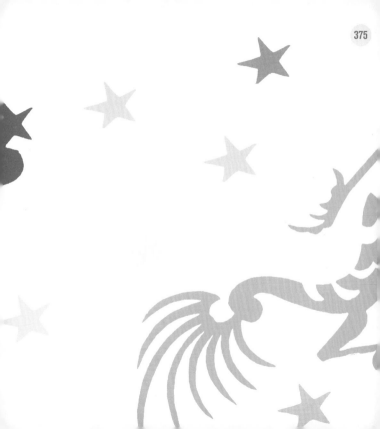

"What did he say?" asked Lien Shu.

"He said that far away, on Ku Mountain, there lives an immortal whose flesh and skin are as white and smooth as snow. He is as fine and delicate as a young girl. It is said that he never eats food but subsides on the air and dew.

He mounts the clouds and rides on the back of dragons, wandering all about the four seas. With his spirit powers he can protect anyone from sickness or decay and ensure a bountiful harvest. This seems to me to be ridiculous and I cannot believe any of it." Lien Shu then told him, "Everything

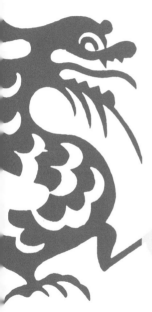

Chien Wu says is true. The blind cannot see elegant shapes and the deaf cannot hear the music of the bells and drums. But blindness and deafness are not just physical, they can also be mental. So it is with yourself. This sage looks upon all the different manifestations of the world as one. Because of him, we are all better for it. Nothing can harm such a person. A great flood could not drown him.

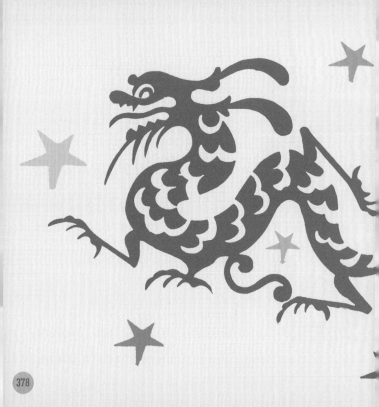

The greatest heat, one that could melt metals and stone, could not harm him. From his very being he could fashion great philosopher kings. Why should he bother with our world?"

CHUANG TZU

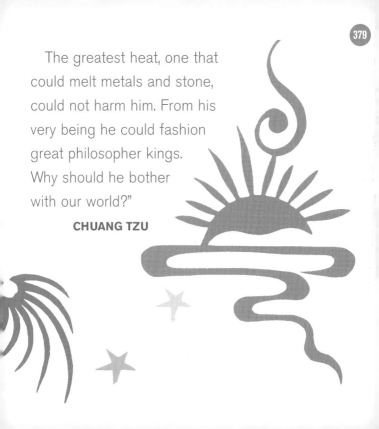

His spirit wise, his essence holy, he illuminates the mysterious and subtle, comprehending the workings of the Real. While still at a distance, he perceives himself and the entire universe as one, as partaking of the same eternal nature.

CHOU SHAO-HSIEN

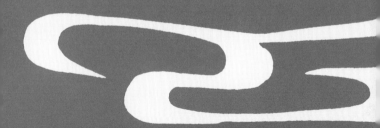

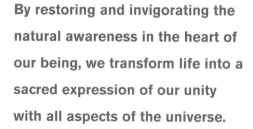

By restoring and invigorating the natural awareness in the heart of our being, we transform life into a sacred expression of our unity with all aspects of the universe.

NI HUA CHING

We are all already Immortals. We only have to recognize ourselves as the true spiritual beings that we are.

We have only to look into the mirror of the soul and see our reflections there, smiling gently back out at us, beckoning us into the deepest expression of God, of the divine, of the Tao. We only have to become who we truly are!

As for recluses famed for such meager attainments as being immune from pillage by wandering soldiery, subduing demons, being invulnerable to poison and disease, being able to travel safely through the mountains beset by savage beasts or to wade streams unharmed by crocodiles and dragons, being immune from epidemics, become invisible when danger threatens–all these are trivial matters, though one needs to be aware of them.

KO HUNG

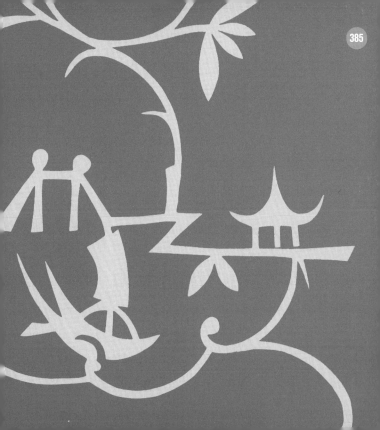

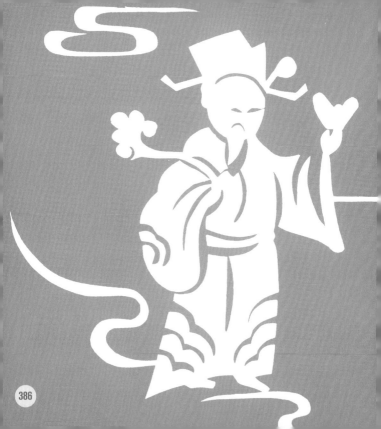

To become an Immortal, to become a sage, to become a wise man or woman, takes a level of commitment not found in the ordinary person. It is not something you can learn in a weekend workshop or from reading a book or watching a video. Teachers can certainly be helpful but it is really one's own self-cultivation that will produce the light that will illuminate your life and help you to realize your own essential nature as being one with the Tao.

You can certainly benefit from the results of doing a spiritual practice in many ways. Heightened sensitivity, emotional balance, psychological insights, greater depth of intuition, a stronger, more healthy lifestyle—all of these can be experienced with just a little work and a little attention to detail.

It is in the details of things that the most spiritual advancement can often be made. In other words, deal with problems while they are still small, and then, if there is something you can't really do anything about, don't let it worry you, don't let it take over your life.

A sage is someone who knows when to be serious and when to be joyous, when to be aggressive and when to yield, when to move forward and when to simply stop and wait.

It is said that each person who attains Immortality carries many of the rest of us along. Traditionally, serious practitioners would retire from the world, but it is important for these times that we do much of our spiritual cultivation in the world. In this way we take society with us as we become more harmonious, more enlightened beings.

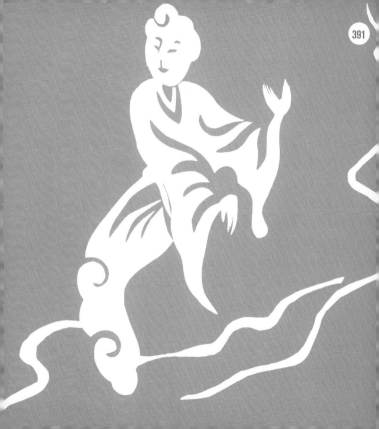

To attain Tao,

It is not necessary

To go to the mountains.

Stay right here,

In the red dust, riding a golden horse–

There is a great practitioner of Tao.

Thus it is said

The mountains only provide quietude.

LU DONG BIN

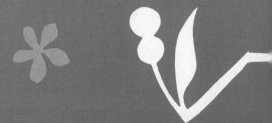

One of the ways we stop ourselves from knowing the Tao is by being too fixed in our thinking. Instead of being like water flowing through a ravine we stop the flow by our own thoughts and attitudes.

Instead of keeping sight of the bigger picture, we get bogged down in the petty details of life that keep us from experiencing our true selves.

The journey of a thousand miles begins with one step. The road to enlightenment begins with each moment.

People may sit until the cushion
is worn through,
But never quite know the real Truth;
Let me tell you about the ultimate Tao:
It is here, enshrined within us.

LU DONG BIN

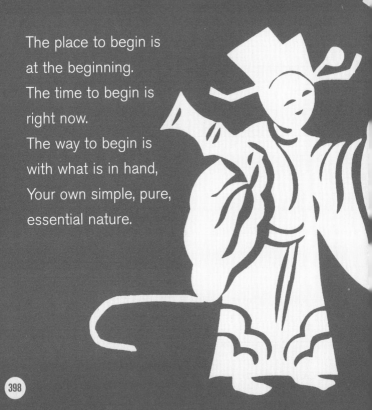

The place to begin is
at the beginning.
The time to begin is
right now.
The way to begin is
with what is in hand,
Your own simple, pure,
essential nature.

The line between confused
human being and sage is,
in reality, a thin and tenuous one.
All it takes is being open to
learning, to growing, to making
mistakes, to confronting our
own fears and ambitions and
a willingness to leap off
into the unknown.

How can we know if we
are on the Way?
Because we have never left it!
How can we know if we are
enlightened or not?
By forgetting what
is ephemeral
and remembering what
is eternal.

The Way of Tao is a simple yet sublime
combination of down-to-earth practicality
and the ability to soar among the clouds
on the backs of dragons!

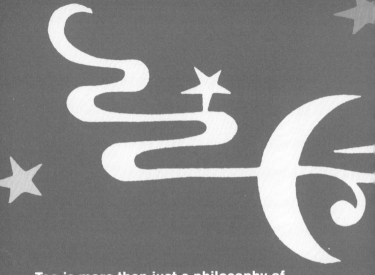

Tao is more than just a philosophy of life. It's a whole way of life, and the only way to realize practical benefits from Tao is to cultivate and practice it.

402

DANIEL REID

The space between heaven and
earth is like a bellows.
It is empty yet never loses its form.
It moves yet keeps on moving.
Many words are not as good
as a few.
Maintain the center.

LAO TZU

Sit quietly and let your
mind empty.
Pay attention to each
passing moment
Then let it go.
Let your breath be
your guide.

Abide in the
eternal moment
And feel yourself
slipping into the
greater Self.
This is the Way of
the Immortals!

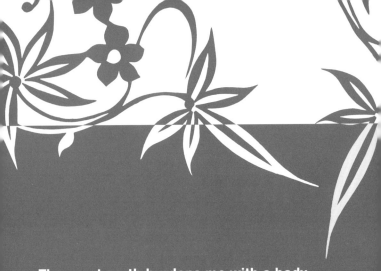

The great earth burdens me with a body,
causes me to toil in life, eases me in old age,
and rests me in death. That which makes my
life good, makes my death good.

CHUANG TZU

We who live our lives in fear of death are ultimately committing ourselves to fear of life itself.

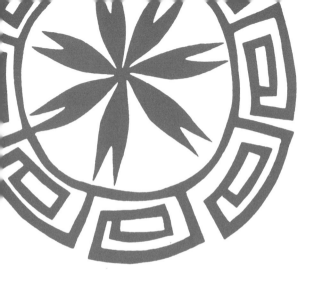

Only he who conquers
himself may be called
a great conqueror.

Those who know that they
have enough are wealthy.
Those who go hold their
place have great power.
Those who do not lose
their place will endure.
To die but not to perish is
to be eternally present.

LAO TZU

It is in that experience of being eternally present that we are able to transcend what we usually think of as time. And in that experiencing, that eternally present moment, death does not exist. Death, as the end of life, has no meaning.

How do I know that in clinging to this life I'm not merely clinging to a dream and delaying my entry into the real world?

CHUANG TZU

Bridle the mind, for it is like a wild horse. It needs to be tamed. First one has to know it is there, running on the plain. Then try to catch it, ride it, lead it by the reins and be watchful of its movements all the time. With firmness, gentleness, and patience, the horse will be tamed and the master known.

HUA CHING NI

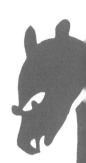

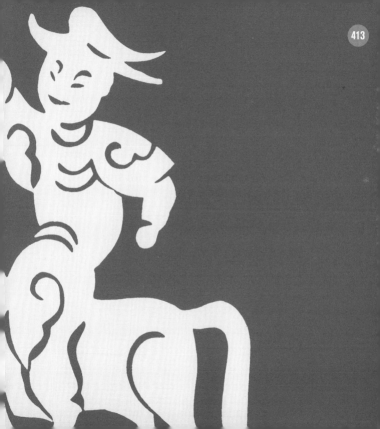

To truly understand who we are
and what we think this life is all
about we must plumb to the very
depths of what we know of as
ourselves, we must allow
ourselves to sink as deeply
as we can in order to reach
that place of surrender, of
acceptance, of true knowledge.

It is then that all book knowledge, all acquired knowledge, all borrowed or stolen knowledge melts away. And in its place is a surety, a sense of safety, or trust. Trust in the Tao, in that eternal cycle of the seasons, of life, death, and rebirth.

Surrender yourself humbly;

Then you can be trusted to care for all things.

Love the world as your own self;

Then you can truly care for all things.

LAO TZU

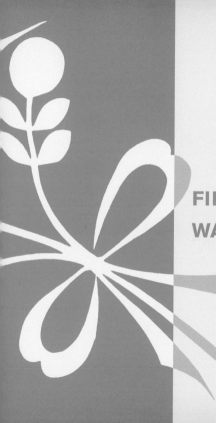

FINDING THE WAY

Once there lived men and women
who were not conscious of their
separation from Tao,
therefore they were
at one with it.

Chuang Tzu describes this kind of person as not minding being poor. They took pride in their achievements. They made no plans. In this way, they could commit an error and not regret it. They could succeed without being proud. In this way, they could climb mountains without fear, enter water without getting wet, and pass through fire without being burned. They slept without dreaming and awoke without anxiety. Their food was simple and their breath was deep.

They did not love life or hate death. When they were born they felt no elation, when they died there was no sorrow. Carefree they came. Carefree they went. That was all. They did not forget their beginning and yet did not seek their end. They accepted all that was given them with delight and when it was gone, they gave it no more thought.

Nowadays, we strive and struggle, never content, always sure there is something greater to achieve, something of greater value and worth if only we can become successful in the eyes of the world. Yet at the end of the day, in the deep of the night, in the first glare of the morning light we feel empty and bereft.

We have lost the Way and are now very far indeed from those ancient men and woman who lived so well and so lightly.

All life is change. Don't hang on to the moment. Let it go and evolve into the next one. Don't become attached to the good times or worry unduly about the bad times.

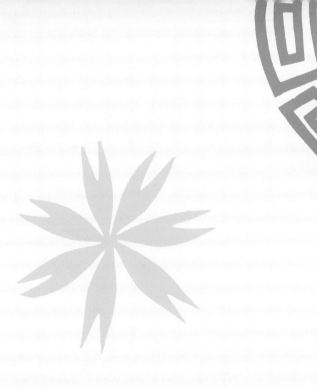

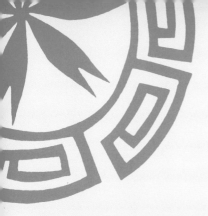

The wheel of life keeps turning,
one day up, the next one down.
By not holding on to the good
times we are better able to deal
with the bad times.

In life, don't look for divisions, but notice, instead, the places of agreement. Don't emphasize differences, instead look for opportunities to share. Don't pay undue attention to your failures but honor your successes, no matter how small.

The Path of Tao gives us ways to cultivate ourselves spiritually, energetically, and emotionally. It gives us specific practices to bring all our varying and vying selves in focus, harmony and the oneness where we truly dwell— the eternal, ever-evolving Tao.

Tao, then, is the Way, as in direction, manner, source, destination, purpose, and process. In discovering and exploring Tao the process and the outcome are one and the same. The Way to the goal, the Way along the Way, the one who is going along the Way—they are all one and the same.

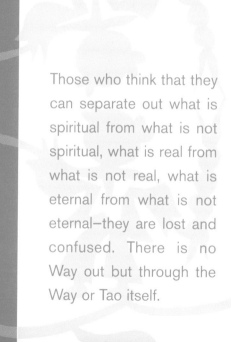

Those who think that they can separate out what is spiritual from what is not spiritual, what is real from what is not real, what is eternal from what is not eternal—they are lost and confused. There is no Way out but through the Way or Tao itself.

Just as there are many different kinds of trees in the forest so too are there many different approaches to the Tao.

All paths are aspects of the one path, all truths are but the one truth, everything that rises must converge. The man or woman of Tao understands this and acts accordingly. For them the past, the present, and the future are all of a piece. They make no distinctions between things, persons, or states of being. In this way they free themselves from the cycle of change and dwell in the infinite Tao.

In the Path of Tao we call spiritual work cultivation. We plant the spiritual seeds into our beings and wait patiently for them to grow. We attend them and water them with our tears of joy and grief and mulch them with the negative experiences of our life. And then, if we are patient enough, we can experience the flowering of our Tao Nature and flourish like a great flower in the sun.

Once there was a great craftsman who fashioned a mulberry leaf out of jade to give to the king. He worked on it for three years and when he was done and it was placed in a bowl along with other mulberry leaves its veins, its shape, its color were so realistic it could not be distinguished from the real ones. The king was so impressed by his work that he immediately appointed him to his court.

When Lieh Tzu heard of this he said:

"If heaven and earth took so long to grow things that it took three years to grow a leaf, there would not be many things with leaves."

Therefore the follower of Tao puts her trust in the unfolding of the Way and not in cunning and skill.

LIEH TZU

By being humble, by not putting on airs, by not having opinions, we can open ourselves to new experiences and attain true knowledge. This is known on the Path of Tao as "leading from behind."

Become quiet,
become humble,
become invisible.
In this way you will
become worthy of
entering the Tao!

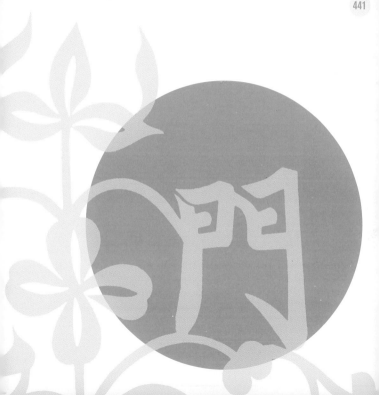

In straw sandals

and a belt of hemp

in a rush raincoat

dangling an old gourd ladle

half like a fisherman

half like a woodcutter

my head like a raspberry patch

and my face like a dump

I'll bear your laughter.

YUN-KAN TZU

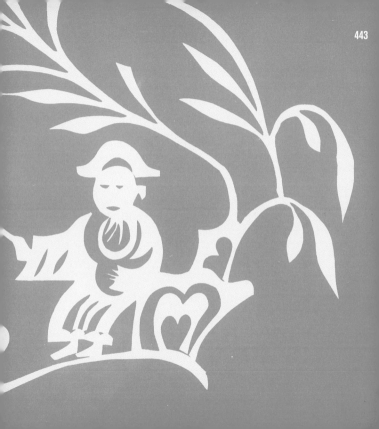

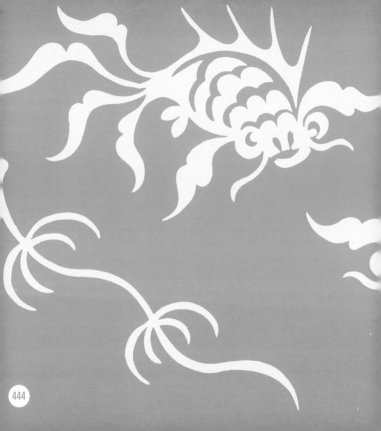

The students of Tao do not want to stand out in the crowd, do not want others to think too highly of them, do not want to draw too much attention to themselves. Rather they would appear humble, even foolish in the eyes of the world. Living a simple, straightforward life is what they seek. Like water, they wish to learn how to flow with the Tao and create themselves anew each moment, in whatever shape or situation they find themselves in.

Following what is sometimes called the Watercourse Way, the men or women of Tao fashion their lives anew in each moment, adapting to every new situation as it evolves. In this way they are not trapped by the past nor bound to the future, but are constantly renewed and reborn in each instant of their lives. They cultivate themselves—spiritually, mentally, and emotionally—and act as though their lives were great works of art and they are both the artist and art itself.

They are open, yielding, soft yet hard, and sensitive to the slightest nuance of what is appropriate action at any given time. In this way they are free from the constrictions of time and fate, beholden only to their own virtue and sense of the great unfolding Tao.

The man or woman of Tao conceals their attainment. When problems come up they resolve them quickly. When people come to them for assistance they give freely.

HUAINANZI

When we seek outwardly
we seek for things we
feel we lack. When
seeking inwardly, we
find fulfillment
within ourselves.

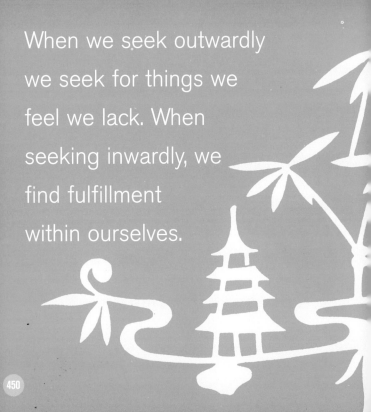

The realized journeyer does not know where she is going. Realizing that all paths lead to the One she travels contentedly.

The most balanced person is not always recognized for what he is; when you look at him, you will not see anything outstanding about him.

HUA CHING NI

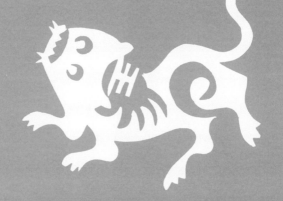

To attain Tao we must become sensitive to the subtle currents of energy in our being—spiritual, physical, and emotional.

The teaching of spiritual alchemy says that when the mind runs off one should gather it in; having gathered it in, then let go of it. After action, seek rest; finding rest, one develops enlightenment. Who says one cannot find tranquility in the midst of clamor and activity?

CHANG SAN FENG

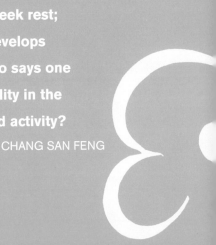

If one is true to one's self and follows its teaching, who need be without a teacher?

CHUANG TZU

Under heaven nothing is more
soft and weaker than water.
Yet for attacking the hard, the
resistant, nothing can surpass it.
The weak can conquer the strong,
The soft can conquer the hard.
Under heaven everyone knows this
Yet no one seems to apply it.

LAO TZU

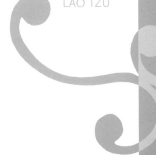

When your work is
done, withdraw,
This is the Way of
Heaven.

LAO TZU

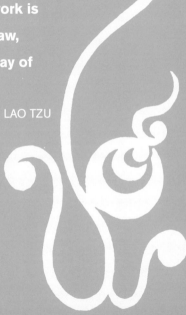

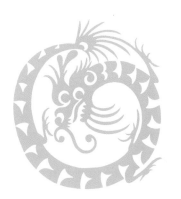

Bibliography

Blofeld, John. *Taoism: The Road to Immortality*. Boston: Shambhala, 1985.

Blofeld, John. *Taoist Mysteries and Magic*. Boulder: Shambhala.

Chan, Alan K. L. *Two Visions of the Way: A Study of the Wang-Pi and the Ho-shang Kung Commentaries on the Lao-Tzu*. New York: State University of New York Press, 1991.

Chen, Ellen M. *The Tao Te Ching: A New Translation with Commentary*. New York: Paragon House, 1989.

Chia, Mantak & Maneewan. *Awaken Healing Light of the Tao*. Huntington, NY: Healing Tao Books, 1993.

Cleary, Thomas, trans. *Further Teachings of Lao-tzu: Understanding the Mysteries*. Boston: Shambhala, 1991.

Cleary, Thomas, trans. *The Tao of Politics*. Boston: Shambhala, 1990.

Cleary, Thomas, trans. *The Taoist Classics*, Vol. 2. Boston: Shambhala, 1986.

Cleary, Thomas, trans. *The Taoist I Ching*. Boston: Shambhala, 1986.

Feng, Gia-Fu and Jane English, trans. *Chuang Tsu: Inner Chapters*. New York: Vintage, 1974.

Feng, Gia-Fu and Jane English, trans. *Lao Tsu: Tao Te Ching*. New York: Alfred A. Knopf, 1972.

Graham, A.C., trans. *The Book of Lieh-tzu: A Classic of Tao*. New York:

Columbia University Press, 1960.

Hinton, David, trans. *The Selected Poems of Li Po*. New York: New Directions, 1996.

Kaltenmark, Max. *Lao Tzu and Taoism*. Stanford, Calif.: Stanford University Press, 1969.

Lu, Ke Yun, Lucy Liao, trans. *The Essence of Qigong*. Eugene, Oregon: The Abode of the Eternal Tao, 1998.

Merton, Thomas. *The Way of Chuang Tzu*. New York: New Directions, 1965.

Ming-Dao, Deng. *365 Tao: Daily Meditations*. San Francisco: HarperSanFrancisco, 1992.

Ming-Dao, Deng. *Everyday Dao: Living with Balance and Harmony*. San Francisco: HarperSanFrancisco, 1996.

Ming-Dao, Deng. *Scholar Warrior*. San Francisco: HarperSanFrancisco, 1990.

Ni, Hua-Ching. *The Gentle Path of Spiritual Progress*. Los Angeles: The Shrine of the Eternal Breath of Tao and College of Tao and Traditional Chinese Healing, 1987.

Ni, Hua-Ching. *Internal Alchemy: The Natural Way to Immortality*. Los Angeles: The Shrine of the Eternal Breath of Tao and College of Tao and Traditional Chinese Healing, 1992.

Ni, Hua-Ching. *Tao: The Subtle Universal Law and the Intergral Way of Life*. Los Angeles: College of Tao and Traditional Chinese Healing, 1979.

Nisker, Wes. *Crazy Wisdom*. Berkeley: Ten Speed Press, 1990.

Reid, Daniel. *The Complete Book of Chinese Health and Healing: Guarding the Three Treasures*. Boston: Shambhala, 1994.

Reid, Daniel. *The Tao of Health, Sex & Longevity: A Modern Practical Guide to the Ancient Way*. New York: Fireside, 1989.

Schipper, Kristofer. *The Taoist Body*. Berkeley: University of California Press, 1993.

Seaton, Jerome P., trans. *The Wine of Endless Life: Taoist Drinking Songs*. Buffalo, NY: White Pine Press, 1985.

Smullyan, Raymond M. *The Tao is Silent*. San Francisco: HarperSanFrancisco, 1977.

Ware, James R., trans. *Alchemy, Medicine & Religion in the China of A.D. 320: The Nei P'ien of Ko Hung*. New York: Dover, 1966.

Watts, Alan, with Al Chung-liang Huang. *Tao: The Watercourse Way*. New York: Pantheon Books, 1975.

Watts, Alan. *Taoism: Way Beyond Seeking*. Boston: Tuttle Publishing, 1997.

Welch, Holmes. *Taoism: The Parting of the Way*. Boston: Beacon Press, 1957.

Wilhelm, Richard, trans. *The Secret of The Golden Flower: A Chinese Book of Life*. New York: Causeway Books, 1975.

Wong, Eva. *Lieh-Tzu: A Taoist Guide to Practical Living*. Boston: Shambhala, 1995.

Yu, Lu K'uan. *Ch'an and Zen Teaching*. York Beach, Maine: Samuel Weiser, 1993.

Author Biography

Solala Towler is a musican, poet, and teacher. He is editor of *The Empty Vessel, A Journal of Contemporary Taoism*, a magazine with an international subscription and base (www.abodetao.com). He is also author of *A Gathering of Cranes: Bringing the Tao to the West* and *Embarking On the Way: A Guide to Western Taoism*. He is an instructor of Taoist meditation and of several styles of *chi gong*. He has taught classes and seminars all over the U.S. and abroad and is currently President of the National Qigong Association* U.S.A.

Solala leads yearly tours to China to study *chi gong*, and visits Taoist temples and sacred mountains. You can email him at solala@abodetao.com or call (001)-541-345-8854.

First published by MQ Publications Limited
12 The Ivories, 6–8 Northhampton St., London, N1 2HY

Library of Congress Cataloging-in-Publication Data
Towler, Solala
   Tao paths to harmony/Solala Towler
      p. cm.
   ISBN: 0-7407-2296-4
   1. Harmony (Philosophy) 2. Tao. I. Title.

BD105.H T68 2002
299.5144–dc21   2001046432

Printed and bound in China